TIME TO SELL?

GUIDE TO SELLING A PHYSICIAN PRACTICE:
VALUE, OPTIONS, ALTERNATIVES

— THIRD EDITION —

By Randy Bauman

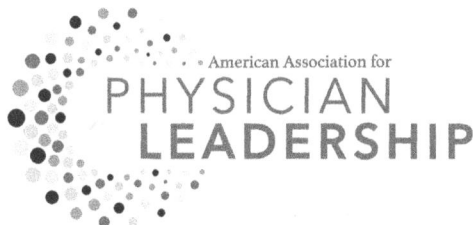

American Association for
PHYSICIAN
LEADERSHIP

13   8 7 6 5 4 3 2 1
Copyedited, typeset, indexed, and printed in the United States of America

PUBLISHER
Nancy Collins

EDITORIAL ASSISTANT
Jennifer Weiss

DESIGN & LAYOUT
Carter Publishing Studio

INDEX
Pamela Reigeluth

COPYEDITOR
Karen Doyle

Table of Contents

Dedication

To my daughter, Arial.
May the bright sun and the gift of knowledge always shine on you.

Acknowledgements

Writing is a cathartic experience. It requires taking the time to put into words, our experiences, observations, and perspectives in a way we rarely are required to do. It forces organization of thoughts, analysis of trends, and consideration of options and alternatives. It requires expressing an opinion. The process made me a better trusted advisor to my clients.

Thanks to Carla Hall for all of her encouragement, suggestions, and world-class proofreading skills (and for driving the truck) during the writing of the first two editions.

Thanks to Angela Herron and Leif Beck for reading the manuscript and providing excellent comments and suggestions that made this a better book.

Thanks to Daryl Demonbreun, my business partner, for always being there.

Thanks to Bob Maier, who took a chance on a green kid and taught him about healthcare.

Thanks to Jon Grimes, who taught me more about physician practices than anyone in spite of his background as a hospital CEO.

Finally, thank you to Nancy Collins at Greenbranch Publishing for her encouragement, support, and suggestions, and to all the folks at Greenbranch who helped make this book a reality.

Randy Bauman
April, 2016

About the Author

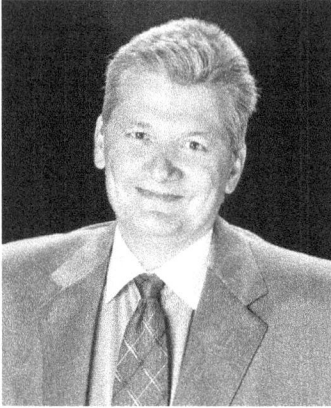

Randy Bauman is president of Delta Health Care (www.deltahealthcare.com) in Franklin, Tennessee. For over 30 years, Randy has advised physician groups and hospitals on the business of physician practice, including group practice development, strategic planning, mergers and acquisitions, group formations, compensation, governance, operations, and practice valuations.

His books, articles, and speeches challenge conventional wisdom and the lemming behavior in healthcare. He is a frequent speaker at Medical Group Management Association (MGMA) and Healthcare Financial Management Association (HFMA) chapters and has presented numerous audio conferences on a diverse range of topics such as The Changing Hospital/Physician Relationship, Reality Check—I'm Not in Control of My Practice, and Disruptive Physicians and How to Deal with Them.

He has been interviewed by and had articles published in numerous healthcare publications, including *The Journal of Medical Practice Management*, *Medical Economics*, *The Physician's Advisory*, *Doctor's Digest*, *Unique Opportunities*, *ACP Observer*, *The Journal of Family Practice*, and *Group Practice Solutions*.

He is a member of the MGMA, the American Health Lawyers Association, and Toastmasters International.

He lives in Mesquite, Nevada, and in his spare time he pursues his passions for travel, photography, and motorcycling. Contact Randy at rb@deltahealthcare.com.

Foreword

Americans receive the best healthcare in the world. Our physicians are superbly trained and committed to giving conscientious, highly specialized care while being personally concerned for patients' welfare. Our hospitals are technological marvels spawned by a huge supply of both financial and human capital.

Still, at least at the doctor level, we just can't seem to get it right. Various social and political forces threaten to kill the will of this most essential healthcare component—the physicians who provide the brains and judgment to diagnose and treat an incredible variety of patient problems.

Having consulted to so many of these fine people for some 37 years, I stand in awe of and feel distress for them. How, I wonder, can so many highly able providers of top-quality care do so much good on an individual basis and yet struggle so much to make their personal and financial lives acceptable? And how can it be that, while physicians in some specialties are highly successful economically, a growing number of others just aren't making it?

Randy Bauman, author of this fine book, can't, of course, answer those overriding questions any better than anyone else. But having known and worked with so many medical practice advisors over the years, I've come to respect his technical abilities and practical judgment in working with medical practices and their physician members. He has seen and dealt with it all, honestly and openly, with (mostly) excellent results for his clients.

One of the issues he's dealt with extensively the past few years is the subject of this book. The idea of selling out was oddly popular back in the mid- and late-1990s because both hospitals and physician practice management companies (PPMCs) were offering what quickly turned out to be foolishly high prices. Randy and I, and indeed almost all medical consultants, went through that period when some doctors sold out "at the top." Not more than a couple of years later, the hospitals and PPMCs discovered their over-generosity and resold many of those practices back at huge losses.

This time around, things are different. While some physicians and groups can command surprisingly high prices, for many other doctors, the economics may or may not be there. Doctors see ever-increasing regulation, decreasing reimbursement, and heavy fixed costs (including malpractice insurance) bearing down on them both financially and emotionally. The situation leads more of them than ever to say, "I just want to get out of the business and simply take care of patients." Selling out is an increasingly popular option, but whether it's for you, and if so how to go about it, is not a simple matter.

Randy has been heavily involved in advising whether doctors should (or can) sell their practices, and if so how to do it and at what price. Reading this book, I can just see and hear Randy giving the "real skinny" in reply to questions about selling out. No book I know of has more direct talk or honest, down-to-earth advice on the subject.

Time to Sell? Guide to Selling a Physician Practice: Value, Options, Alternatives deals with all the aspects of the urge to sell. It starts right in with the first—and major—question: Why do you want to sell, and is such an action the right thing for you? The book ends by coming back to that basic question, forthrightly discussing your other options for much the same reason—that selling out must fit the doctor personally even more so than on the technical issues. I've worked with Randy enough times to know how much the personally "right" result matters to him.

In between these two bookends, he offers sophisticated advice in a down-to-earth, understandable way. I've struggled sometimes to explain ideas like the discounted cash flow approach in helping set an asking price, but—having been through it literally hundreds of times—Randy makes it understandable. Then in Chapters 6 through 9, he takes it past the valuation question by coaching how to make the deal. After all, having a price and negotiating a result are two vastly different matters, each calling for special attention.

And to help ensure that the reader gets it, *Time to Sell? Guide to Selling a Physician Practice: Value, Options, Alternatives* lists specific takeaway points and provides checklists at the end of each chapter.

Randy is not an attorney, and although I am, it's good that he isn't. While you absolutely need a well-qualified lawyer to finalize the sale, I've seen lawyers kill too many desirable medical practice deals. *Time to Sell? Guide to Selling a Physician Practice: Value, Options, Alternatives* recognizes the legal formalities but, more importantly, serves as a practical guide to help you reach the best possible results for you.

You, after all, have to make the right judgments—not your lawyer, consultant, or other advisors. By reading this book carefully, you should feel well-prepared to deal with an issue that is rising more quickly than you may realize.

Leif C. Beck, JD, CHBC
Founder and Former Publisher of *The Physician's Advisory* and *Group Practice Success* Newsletters, and Medical Management Consultant

Introduction

Trends, like horses, are easier to ride in the direction they are going.

John Naisbitt

The cycle of hospital employment of physician practices continues to move around the circle. When I completed the first edition of this book in August 2008, I noted: "the trend is unmistakable—physicians continue to sell their practices at a feverish pace. In my role as a practice consultant, working with both hospitals and physician practices, I can tell you this trend is taking on tsunami proportions."

When Nancy Collins at Greenbranch and I first discussed a second edition, I was pleased to hear that the sales of the first edition had been steady for three years—meaning the book had exhibited what publishers call "shelf life." Why change a good thing? Well, much had changed.

That is the case again now, in 2015, as I complete the third edition. Hospital employment of physicians follows a predictable cycle and this cycle now seems destined to go full circle in many situations.

The passage of the Patient Protection and Affordable Care Act in March 2010 accelerated the sales of physician practices. While some experts credited (or blamed) the demise of private practice on health reform, the trend had been present for some time.

For the rest of 2010 and early 2011, the buzzword *de jour* was "Accountable Care Organizations" or ACOs—that is until the Centers for Medicare & Medicaid Services issued its proposed regulations in the spring of 2011, which chilled the enthusiasm greatly.

But the fact is, healthcare does have to change. The quote above from management guru John Naisbitt illustrates that trends tend to take on a life of their own. There is a bit of lemming behavior in most business trends, and those of us in the healthcare industry saw a similar trend of hospitals buying physician practices unfold and reach feverish proportions in the 1990s. The existence of a clear trend does not ensure the success of the underlying strategy, and I warned in the first edition that caution was in order.

The second edition addressed the continuing evolution in the physician practice marketplace and those changes continue. The second edition addressed the predictable increase in prices for physician practices as competition heated up and the accelerated payment for intangible assets and goodwill. Controversy on how practices can and should be valued, with prominent experts holding near-polar-opposite opinions on both sides, also was explored.

This third edition has been significantly expanded to reflect that while these trends continue, the marketplace has reached its zenith in some areas. The prices being paid and the economic losses being incurred are simply not financially viable. The compensation being offered will lead to the demise of more than a few hospital CEOs and physician practice leaders because the deals now being structured ultimately will be financially unsustainable. As noted above, there is a distinct, quite-predictable cycle of hospital employment of physicians. What I am seeing in the marketplace, coupled with this history, motivated me to add a new chapter, Chapter 1, "The Cycle of Physician Employment," which should serve as a ready reference guide to readers.

This edition was updated from the previous editions to reflect the most current information. If you are considering selling your practice but are skeptical, you should spend some time reading Chapter 1. It will give you a feel for where the industry is and the huge challenges you may face if you sell and it doesn't work out. Unless your retirement is imminent, selling your practice at this stage in the cycle of physician employment should be pursued only after carefully considering a possible exit strategy.

My original query in 2008, when I completed the first edition, was whether hospital/physician partnerships would survive. That question has become even more important today.

The original purpose of this guide remains the same: "to walk physicians and practice managers through the process of objectively evaluating a practice and determining whether selling is the right option." The practical advice, war stories, pitfalls, questions, and checklists will help you no matter which side you find yourself.

I do not think private practice is dead, but the changing climate of healthcare will make it challenging for private practice to survive. I see more and more physicians disillusioned with private practice; they are reconciled to selling or merging their practice and making the best deal they can. At the same time, hospitals' success or failure in this wave of employment has not been determined. Success will be driven by the hospitals' willingness and ability to transcend typical hospital-centric thinking and try new models and approaches. There is no simple answer that applies to all practices and all situations. Take some time to consider all the options presented in this book, then decide what works best for you.

CHAPTER 1

The Cycle of Physician Employment

Those who fail to study history are doomed to repeat it. Anonymous

The 1990s saw a feeding frenzy of hospitals snapping up physician practices, paying huge acquisition prices, and guaranteeing the doctors cushy salaries. Within a few short years, hospitals were losing an average of $100,000 per physician annually and the acquisition binge became a divestiture binge. The resulting implosion was monumental. Long-tenured CEOs were dismissed, hospital debt ratings were lowered, and some hospitals had to be sold as a result of the huge losses sustained. Physicians found themselves having to reestablish themselves in private practice and facing the reality that their future incomes were going to decrease.

The trend of hospitals buying physician practices reemerged in the mid- to late-2000s as, once again, hospital acquisition and employment of physician practices became a common hospital strategy. At first, hospitals seemed more cautious, deliberately avoiding some of the strategies that had led to failure in the 1990s. Acquisition prices were generally void of goodwill and intangible asset purchases and compensation plans avoided guaranteed salaries, relying instead on productivity-based models.

This acquisition trend continues today, but the past few years have seen the reemergence of the transaction structures that led to the implosion in the 1990s: increasingly higher practice purchase prices (including intangible assets and, in some cases, goodwill) and guaranteed compensation structures without concomitant productivity standards.

Has the reemergence of these two factors planted the seeds for another implosion?

The initial hospital strategy of acquiring and employing physicians to maintain or grow market share and assuring an adequate supply of physicians to support their mission has shifted. The post-Affordable Care Act (ACA) strategy is to develop the critical mass requisite for large, clinically integrated networks. Many hospitals believe these networks are necessary for participation in risk contracting, population health management, and accountable care payment models that government and commercial payors are attempting to establish.

As losses on employment of physicians mount, the question becomes twofold: 1) will the expected "new money" from these risk-based payment models and population health management arrive in time, and 2) will it be enough to sustain the losses? The jury is still out, but the losses represent an increasing risk to physicians looking to sell their practices as well as to the hospitals and health systems purchasing them.

AWARENESS AND ACTION

Physicians seeking to sell their practices and become hospital employees should make themselves aware that the hospital acquisition and employment of physicians seems to be repeating the same cycle we saw in the 1990s. In its basic form, the cycle has three phases: Phase 1: Acquisition, Phase 2: Operational Development, and Phase 3: Restructuring/Divestiture. This cycle is illustrated in Figure 1-1.

Assessing where the local healthcare market or hospital is within this cycle can provide valuable insight to physicians who are considering the sale of their practice, as well as those already employed, because it provides insight into likely future events.

Signs indicate that this cycle, which went full circle in the 1990s, is doing so again and could be heading toward a collision course with economic reality. The Medical

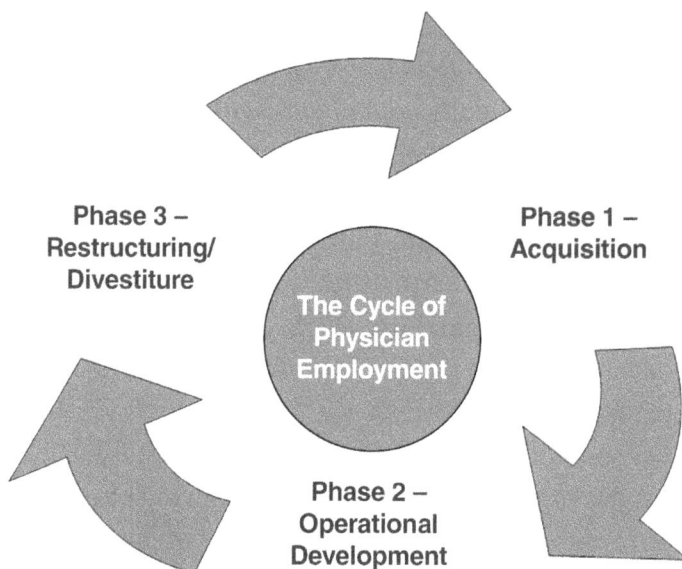

Phase 3 –
Restructuring/
Divestiture

Phase 1 –
Acquisition

The Cycle of
Physician
Employment

Phase 2 –
Operational
Development

FIGURE 1-1. The Cycle of Physician Employment

Specialty Net Loss per FTE Physician*	2014	2015
Family Medicine	$192,213	$110,529
Internal Medicine	$249,339	$136,518
OB-GYN	$412,091	$252,635
Cardiology	$624,150	$388,260
Orthopedic Surgery	$356,582	$333,665
General Surgery	$465,184	$276,750
Average	$383,093	$249,726

FIGURE 1-2. * Median loss excluding financial support per FTE physician for hospital/integrated delivery systems by specialty. 2014 data from the Medical Group Management Association 2014 Cost Survey for Single-Specialty Practices; 2015 data from the Medical Group Management Association 2015 Cost and Revenue Report.

Group Management Association (MGMA) statistics on the median losses per physician for hospital/integrated delivery systems by specialty for 2014 and 2015 (2013 and 2014 data) are illustrated in Figure 1-2.

It is difficult to imagine that losses of this magnitude are sustainable. Moreover, the agencies that rate hospital bonds have long memories of the debacle that ensued in the 1990s. My company personally saw large and unceremonious waves of divestitures of physician practices as losses from physician employment mounted and borrowing costs were affected.

In addition, as noted above, it's not known whether "new money" will be injected into the reimbursement system and whether that money will benefit physicians. Many of these incentive payment systems are budget neutral, meaning there will be winners and losers.

So far, the track record of the Pioneer Accountable Care Organizations (ACOs) for Medicare created under the ACA has been less than impressive. Of the 32 Pioneer ACOs that were created, one-third generated no savings at all and 70% of the savings that were generated were generated by three systems, all in the Boston area.

Perhaps even worse was the diminishing return from these initiatives; the savings in year two were half of the savings in year one, and downside risk hasn't even been factored into the equation yet. While many hospitals and hospital systems are "all-in" on this strategy, the question must be raised as to whether a hospital, which is inherently a huge cost center, is the logical place for elimination of unnecessary care, which is the cornerstone of these coordinated care and population health management initiatives.

Some hospital systems have or will figure it out, but many won't. It's a huge gamble. While hospitals expect to lose money employing physicians, as the cycle unfolds, they typically find the losses to be much higher than anticipated. This is usually the result of failed implementation, the generous compensation offered to newly acquired employed physicians, and declining physician productivity. The need for additional management and information technology infrastructure emerges and, coupled with revenue cycle issues, the losses increase even more.

The "bet" is that the odds will change, that the new payment models will produce increased per-unit revenue. And if that fails to materialize, and the initial indicators aren't good, the losses could quickly become unsustainable.

WHERE IS THE HOSPITAL INDUSTRY IN THIS CYCLE?

Most hospitals are somewhere in the late stages of the Phase 2, the Operational Development Phase. While they may continue to acquire practices, most hospitals are struggling to evolve their operational and management infrastructure in order to realize cost efficiencies and to engage physician employees in governance.

Unfortunately, these activities—trying to gain cost efficiencies and engage physicians in governance—while necessary, aren't likely to solve the economic issues. In 30 years of working with physician practices, I can say with certainty that the economic problems are unlikely to be solved on the operating cost side. The issues are almost always on the revenue side—provider productivity and the revenue cycle (billing, collections, payor contracts, and reimbursement rates)—or with the level of physician compensation itself.

While engaging physicians in governance is almost universally touted as a key tenet of a successful integrated network, the harsh reality is that this "governance," generally because of legal restrictions, usually comes with little or no authority. In fact, it is often no more than a feeble and transparent attempt to co-opt physician leadership to the hospital side in economic discussions. Rarely are physicians (or employees of any kind for that matter) willing or able to abide personal financial sacrifice for the good of an organization, no matter how much they are engaged in its operations. When was the last time you saw the CEO of a hospital agree to a 20% pay cut for the good of the organization?

In the later stages of the Operational Development Phase, the hospital begins to experience two other characteristics that inevitably lead to Phase 3, the Restructuring/Divestiture Phase: reorganization and "leakage."

Reorganization usually includes reshuffling or replacement of management and other changes in the organizational structure. During this stage, especially in large organizations, services such as staffing, information technology (IT), billing, and collections are outsourced to third parties. Consultants are brought in to assess the organization and a "redesign" of the compensation plan begins.

All of these efforts are driven by management's desire to "do something"—usually about the financial losses, although this is generally not explicitly stated. The management often uses the consultants' findings and compensation redesign as cover to try to affect changes—usually physician compensation changes (read "reductions")—that would not have been palatable in the earlier phases.

"Leakage" refers to the departure of physicians who, for whatever reason, have determined that employment with the network simply doesn't work for them. Naturally, the greatest motivation for physicians' departure is economic. Reductions in compensation are never palatable and whether such reductions are implemented under the guise of compensation plan redesign or simply happen because of pre-existing contract terms or negotiation of new contracts doesn't matter. Economic motivation trumps. There are other reasons for physician departures, most notably the loss of control over the basic operation of the practice.

A noteworthy generational difference arises here. Older physicians with prior experience in private practice are more likely to have issues with loss of control and the meetings and bureaucracy that come with being employed by larger organizations. Younger physicians are not as bothered by these things because their experience lacks perspective on the financial risk of private practice and the autonomy and responsibility that goes with it.

Knowing and understanding where the hospital or health system in your market is in this cycle is a key component of using the contents of this book, whether you are considering the sale of your practice or previously sold your practice and are disenchanted and looking for other options such as a return to private practice.

While, as noted above, most hospitals are in the late stages of Phase 2, Operational Development, some have entered the early stages of Phase 3, Restructuring and Divestiture, whether they know it or not. Both my company and my (friendly) competitors are seeing leakage and a small but increasing number of unhappy physicians going back into independent practice. Paradoxically, some hospitals are in the early stages of Phase 1, Acquisition, and are just beginning to acquire and employ physician practices. It may be a few years before they reach the later stages of Phase 2.

Some hospitals have successful networks of employed physicians, and a handful leaving to go back into private practice will not materially affect the viability of the network. Others may collapse from the sheer weight of the financial losses, CEO firings, bond rating declines, or from the mass departure of disillusioned physicians who have lost both confidence and interest in the business model.

It is said that healthcare is local, and that is true. Each market is different, but a careful examination of the current situation in your market is in order. An accurate assessment of where your hospital is in this cycle will give you valuable insight into the future and might aid you in both your decision making and negotiating strategy.

The rest of this chapter provides a more detailed description of the characteristics of each phase of this cycle to help you make this assessment.

Phase 1—Acquisition

Hospitals enter into the acquisition phase through many different paths. Some hospitals are forced into physician employment by the physicians themselves, as physicians seek income stability and shelter from day-to-day management responsibilities.

In other cases, physician employment is driven by the hospital's strategic planning process, which often includes a tenet to assure market access by establishing a strong and loyal primary care base. The ACA's provisions that encouraged development of ACOs led many hospitals to conclude that, strategically, they needed a network of physicians to clinically integrate in anticipation of these alternate payment models.

In still other cases, changes in Medicare reimbursement threatened the revenue base of many specialists, which led to a full-scale rush to "lock in" compensation at historical rates (or, more appropriately, historical rates plus a healthy increase) through hospital employment.

Whatever the motivation, Phase 1 is characterized by rapid acquisition, often with little time or thought given to development of the proper infrastructure to operate the employed practices. This is the phase where many mistakes are made that haunt the employed physician network for years to come and, in some cases, sow the seeds for its demise.

Physicians who are considering selling their practice to a hospital that is in this phase are in the "sweet spot." Contract terms and compensation are more negotiable at this stage because the move toward standardization that comes in the later stages of a large network's natural evolution hasn't emerged yet. At this stage, the drive is often to do whatever needs to be done to "get the deal done." In competitive markets, prices hospitals offer often include intangible assets and even goodwill, whereas hospitals in noncompetitive markets will generally eschew these items and only offer to acquire furniture, fixtures, and equipment.

Likewise, compensation plans and models typically aren't standardized at this phase, so while compensation will still need to meet the confines of fair market value and commercial reasonableness (See Chapter 6) compensation offers tend to be more aggressive and compensation tends to be higher. Compensation models are less structured and often vary widely, even between physicians in the same specialty employed by the same hospital.

Lack of a coherent alignment strategy is common in this phase. Responding to physician requests for employment and fear of losing key practices to competitors sows the seeds of acquisitions with ultimately unsustainable transaction structures, including high practice acquisition values and compensation structures. *Take the money and run is the best lesson for physicians fortunate enough to stumble into this situation, but recognize the model may not be sustainable, so have a pre-planned exit strategy if it doesn't work out.*

At this phase, operating losses are almost universally present, but hospitals often have difficulty accurately quantifying the extent of the losses. Hospital finance departments initially lack the resources necessary to quickly and accurately establish meaningful financial reporting for an entirely foreign business line. We've seen hospitals unable to provide separate income statements for physician practices a year or more after beginning to employ physicians.

Physician billing is almost always an issue at this stage as well. Basic revenue cycle processes such as charge capture and claims filing are often mismanaged. Consolidation of multiple and often disparate billing systems or the use of hospital billing departments almost always results in disaster. Use of outside billing companies has a mixed record of success as well, because they are being asked to perform in a highly disorganized and volatile environment.

Hospitals report revenue on an accrual basis (Chapter 8), which means their income statements reflect an estimate of what will be collected. With little history on which to base these estimates, coupled with inexperienced hospital billing personnel or outside billing companies, the actual collections are often much less than what was originally estimated. This leads to inaccurate income statements until there is sufficient history to accurately estimate revenue.

Other seeds of destruction that often are planted at this phase include over-reliance on hospital services such as human resources and finance.

Phase 2—Operational Development

Phase 2 is generally characterized by evolving the operation of standalone physician offices to a more consolidated and standardized group practice platform. This sounds easy, but in reality often takes several years and overlaps dramatically with the late stages of Phase 1 acquisitions.

As the size of the network grows, the reliance on hospital services in areas such as human resources and finance becomes stressed. Usually a senior management position is created and filled by someone experienced in physician practice management. Power struggles between hospital and physician practice management are common and more often than not there is turnover at this position during the early years.

In the past, as losses became more apparent to hospital management and the hospital board, they often considered provider-based billing. While this tactic was outlawed, in most situations, as part of the Bipartisan Budget Act of 2015, it allowed the hospital to convert its employed physician offices to departments of the hospital for Medicare purposes. By meeting certain criteria, the hospital could bill Medicare under the Part A (the hospital side) for the facility fee component of, for example, an office visit, and Medicare Part B (the physician side) for the professional services of the physicians. While the reimbursement under Part B was reduced, the aggregate reimbursement increase is generally in the 20% range.

The downside was that patients received two bills for a simple physician office visit and their out-of-pocket costs would often increase, resulting in patient dissatisfaction and discontent—most of which was directed at the physicians and their office staff.

Another significant downside was that *every* Medicare office visit was billed using the hospital's billing system because the facility portion was billed and paid under Medicare Part A. These small charges were quickly subsumed into the massive hospital billing system and, because of the relatively small dollar amounts involved, became difficult to track and evaluate from a collection standpoint. Measuring true performance on the actual collections on these charges was often impossible.

In many cases, the shift to provider-based billing was a public relations nightmare for the hospital. We saw some hospitals forced to reverse this practice in the face of community opposition and others avoid it altogether in anticipation of opposition.

Although existing provider-based billing is grandfathered under the Bipartisan Budget Act of 2015, the recent elimination of provider-based billing for new off-campus locations may impact the value hospitals are willing to pay for physician practices and will place even more pressure on hospitals already suffering under the weight of losses on employed physician practices.

As Phase 2 evolves, disparate operational processes are moved toward standardization and consolidation. Examples include billing, electronic health records (EHRs), and financial reporting. Office site autonomy is further eroded as hospitals attempt staffing consolidation, and cross-training and policies and procedures become more standardized. Additional infrastructure IT is often added. Benchmarking and financial reporting are standardized. Physician governance across the entire employed network is generally implemented.

As the accuracy of financial reporting and performance benchmarking are improved, most hospitals are unpleasantly surprised that operating losses are much higher than previously forecasted or reported. Such losses are almost always traceable to the revenue side of the equation: physician productivity and revenue cycle issues and the levels of physician compensation established through the acquisition negotiations in Phase 1. Physician productivity, once measurable, is often lower than anticipated, but the decline was often masked by inaccurate or incomplete data.

Basic billing and collection functions such as insurance verification, collection of copayments, and establishment and enforcement of patient financial policies, which are almost always lacking in the earlier stages, are shored up. Hospitals almost universally assert their payor contracts are superior to independent physician practices, but even this is generally found not to be the case.

While the losses are almost always traceable to the revenue side, hospitals almost always focus on the cost side. Having failed to learn the old Tom Peters adage that your ability to cut overhead is limited but your ability to grow revenue is unlimited; hospitals generally focus on cutting costs.

The final step in Phase 2 is usually consolidation. Independent physician practices are generally run in a very cost-efficient manner. The same can't be said for hospitals. Generally the first step in hospital cost-cutting is to combine previously cost-effective and efficient services at the practice level into a consolidated operating environment. This consolidation generally doesn't always include consolidation into one large physician office facility, but sometimes it does.

This consolidation step usually focuses on consolidation of business functions. My favorite is the central billing office or CBO. Consciously sending the people who know the patients to a CBO with an offsite location and phone number is a recipe for failure. In my 30 years in consulting with physician practices, I have rarely seen a

CBO that improves collections or reduces costs—but that doesn't stop every hospital from trying. Another favorite of mine is consolidation of the scheduling function; the results are usually the same as with the CBO.

As Phase 2 reaches its late stages, hospitals generally begin to recognize the need for restructuring, and often wholesale change is in the offing. This is also where many independent-minded physicians begin to feel discontented and start to fantasize about regaining their independence.

Phase 3—Restructuring and Divestiture

Phase 3 usually begins as a frenetic attempt to reduce operating losses and restructure the employed physician network into the viable long-term component of its business strategy. Hospitals rarely enter Phase 3 with the focus of divestiture, but that is sometimes the outcome.

The first step in the restructuring process usually involves bringing in an outside consultant to assess everything in the organization, from management to operations to strategy. The results of this assessment vary widely based on the situation. Sometimes it results in firing of the senior practice management team which in some cases is warranted, but in many others is merely scapegoating.

Standardization of physician employment contracts, if not previously undertaken, is often tackled at this stage. In many situations, the term of the physician employment contracts are at or near their expiration anyway, and the expectation of reimbursement increases tied to nonproductivity incentives as expected new payment models emerge opens the door for restructuring compensation.

We see intense effort being put into developing restructured compensation models in anticipation of population health management initiatives by payors. The problem is that, in most cases, these incentives haven't been defined. Most nonproductivity incentives by payors involve "bonuses" from shared savings or for meeting certain coordination of care, outcomes, cost reductions, and compliance with evidence-based medicine guidelines.

One interesting sidelight to these "bonuses" or "new money" is an emerging debate over how it will actually be divided between the hospital and its employed physicians. The physicians assert they are the ones doing the extra work, changing their practice patterns, and (sometimes) foregoing productivity in order to meet these new guidelines, and should therefore be entitled to the financial benefits.

Of course, the hospital perspective tends to be, although unspoken, that it is already subsidizing physician compensation and absorbing huge operating losses in developing the systems and technology supporting these new payor initiatives, and it should be entitled to a substantial portion of this "new money" as a way to "pay back" or otherwise reduce the ongoing operating losses from the employed physician network.

Restructuring also can involve further consolidation of management services and revenue cycle functions, such as coding and billing as well as IT. Previous consolidation undertaken in Phase 2 is often reconsidered, this time on a broader scale in the case of multi-hospital systems across a region or even an entire hospital system. This is usually done in the name of cost efficiency and standardization.

All of these efforts—assessment, management turnover, compensation restructuring, further changes in governance, and additional consolidation—are primarily motivated by a desire to do two things: reduce the level of losses from the employment of physicians and buy time.

At this stage, senior hospital management is usually under intense pressure from its governing board, the system corporate office or bond rating agencies, banks holding senior debt or, in the case of publicly traded companies, Wall Street, to improve financial performance from employing physicians.

As this phase reaches its later stages, the result is sometimes a deliberate divestiture of underperforming practices or reductions in physician compensation that leave physicians looking for other options. Those physicians who are disgruntled enough begin to explore options and make the difficult choice to try to make a go of it on their own by returning to independent private practice.

Often, leaving is not that simple. Leaving hospital employment and returning to private practice is often limited by contractual terms such as restrictive covenants and noncompete clauses. Depending on the specific contract terms, such departures may require the approval of the hospital employer, and such approval will likely preclude affiliation or sale to a competing hospital or large medical group. Divorces can get messy, and sometimes marriages last beyond their time because of such considerations.

Physicians interested in exploring independence at this stage in the cycle may find the navigation of any legal and financial hurdles easier. The hospital's drive to dramatically reduce losses removes barriers to departure fairly quickly. In the late 1990s, for example, we saw some hospital systems essentially give the physicians back their practices. In some cases, hospitals paid physicians severance to terminate their contracts early and paid for consulting fees to support the physicians going back on their own—all in the interest of getting the losses off their books as soon as possible.

A final interesting sidelight of hospitals experiencing physicians returning to private practice is that hospitals almost always try to keep such departures as low profile as possible—almost as though they fear that widespread knowledge of disgruntled physicians leaving will create a stampede for the door. Based on what happened the last time the industry experienced this cycle, you can't help but wonder if the time will come when hospitals will welcome that stampede.

WHERE DOES THIS LEAVE US?

Is the cycle described above the fate of every hospital system that employs physicians? No. Some hospitals and hospital systems have and will continue to have long-tenured successful physician employment models. They have or will figure it out. Others, as noted, are just getting started and their history hasn't been written.

Determining where your hospital is in this cycle and assessing its ability to attain and retain success is key. The outline above and the checklist at the end of this chapter should provide insight to help you make this judgment in your market situation. My company is currently seeing hospitals in all three phases of this cycle, making these decisions and following these paths. We and other firms like ours are seeing unhappy and disgruntled physicians leaving hospital employment at a pace not seen since the late 1990s. While I don't think we'll see the total demise of physician employment that we saw in the late 1990s, there will most certainly be casualties.

If you are considering selling your practice to a hospital, I encourage you to pay particular attention to Chapter 7 on structuring the deal.

In addition, there are other options discussed in Chapter 11. No one model will survive, and what works will vary widely market by market and physician by physician.

THE CYCLE OF PHYSICIAN EMPLOYMENT
ASSESSMENT CHECKLIST

Check the traits currently present in the hospital's employed physician network in each phase listed below. Generally, the area where you stop making checkmarks will indicate the phase in which your hospital is currently operating its employed physician network and how far it is into that phase.

Phase 1—Acquisition

❑ No formal or communicated acquisition/employment strategy

❑ Few employed physicians

❑ Little or no experience in employing physicians

❏ Flexibility and wide variances in compensation and employment contract terms
❏ Little or no physician practice management infrastructure
❏ Little or no physician engagement in governance
❏ Multiple billing systems at practice level
❏ Hospital departments providing services such as finance, HR, IT

Phase 2—Operational Development

❏ Base of employed physicians (non-hospital-based) with at least 1–3 years tenure
❏ Consolidation of billing and EHR onto common software platform
❏ Hiring or presence of senior physician practice management personnel
❏ Implementation of or functioning physician governance
❏ Implementation or moving toward operational standardization
❏ Moving toward standardization of physician compensation model
❏ Little flexibility in contract terms—standardization of employment contracts
❏ Staffing consolidation and cross-training
❏ Centralization of operating functions such as billing
❏ Network operating costs being allocated to practice level

Phase 3—Restructuring and Divestiture

❏ Concerns expressed on operating losses of physician practices
❏ Outside consultants engaged in practice assessments and performance improvement
❏ Turnaround plans or performance improvement plans
❏ Compensation plan restructuring
❏ Turnover of physician practice management
❏ Use of interim or outside physician practice management
❏ Bond rating downgrades
❏ Hospital C-suite turnover
❏ Physicians leaving the network to return to private practice
❏ Outsourcing of operating functions such as billing and nonclinical staffing
❏ Consolidation of operating functions at corporate or systemwide level

CHAPTER 2

Why Sell?

I always have to remind myself that it's never as good as it seems on the best days and never as bad as it seems on the worst days. That's how I keep my perspective. ANONYMOUS PHYSICIAN

A medical practice is a small business, and running a small business, especially in medicine, has become increasingly complex. Regulatory compliance, declining and uncertain reimbursement, restrictions on ancillary services, physician shortages and rapidly increasing starting salaries, and rising malpractice premiums are just some of the things that seem to be conspiring to make private practices difficult to sustain. No wonder the trend of practices selling out to hospitals has been proceeding at a steady pace for over 10 years.

We will look at some of these issues in more detail below. Before we do, however, you should be aware that if you are considering the sale of your practice at the time of this writing, 2015, you are late to the game. As discussed in Chapter 1, the cycle of physician employment is quite advanced in most markets. That means it is likely that the potential universe of hospital partners has some fairly extensive experience in employing physicians. How are they doing? Are the employed physicians happy with their employment arrangements?

In most situations, hospitals will get mixed reviews: some physicians love being employed, some are miserable. As noted in Chapter 1, many markets with advanced employed physician networks are experiencing some "leakage"—a small but nonetheless steady stream of physicians seeking to return to private practice.

An interesting facet of this leakage is that hospitals usually are loathed to talk about it. It's almost like they don't want the word to get out for fear of starting a stampede for the door. But there are few secrets in most medical communities and you should pay particular attention to any announced departures of physicians from hospital employment. Pay attention to rumors too; terminations often come with confidentiality and other provisions that may legally limit what a departed physician can disclose publicly. Don't be shy about investigating and asking questions, as the additional information and insight you gain will be a valuable part of your ultimate decision.

Let's get back to the factors that typically drive physicians to consider selling.

HEALTHCARE REFORM

The passage of the Patient Protection and Affordable Care Act (ACA) in March 2010 hastened sales of physician practices. While many want to tie the trend to healthcare reform, as noted above, the trend had been proceeding at a feverish pace long before most of us had ever heard of Barack Obama.

Most experts agree that the underpinnings of healthcare reform—lower costs, improved access, and higher quality—are laudable goals. Many physicians, however, tell me they don't understand how they are expected to provide higher quality at lower cost while administrative costs and taxes increase. Physicians have been and continue to be largely unorganized and easy targets for cost-cutting by both government and private payors.

The promise that healthcare reform would provide access to health insurance for an additional 25 million uninsured turned out to be true. Unfortunately, for both providers and patients alike, the term "insurance" didn't turn out to be what many expected. A vast majority of this "new" health insurance coverage turned out to be high-deductible plans, providing providers and patients with insurance coverage for major health issues but often not a plan that actually pays for most routine care.

Many physicians already have full practices and found that these high-deductible plans actually decreased cash flow while making it more difficult to monitor and collect patient balances. Many plans limit or even eliminate coverage for office visits subject to the simple copayment most physician offices had become used to collecting and instead apply office visit charges to the patient's deductible. This leaves the physician's staff responsible not only for collecting 100% of the allowable charge directly from the patient, but also having to navigate and understand the literally dozens of varying plan terms and provisions.

My personal plan, for example, allows two office visits per year and after that, the cost of office visits are applied to a large deductible. How can a small physician practice possibly understand and manage such complexity from what used to be a simple collection of a copay? The days of physician practices simply collecting copayments from patients largely are gone, increasing the complexity of billing and collections and further impacting revenue.

As discussed below, there is an increasing shortage of newly trained physicians, and many are wondering where the physician capacity to treat these newly insured patients is going to come from. It now appears that the shortage will be addressed to an increasing extent by the expanded use of nurse practitioners, physician assistants, and other nonphysician providers. This trend is also unmistakable—20 states now allow nurse practitioners to practice without physician supervision.

The bad news is that the issues of reimbursement cuts, regulation, and malpractice costs weren't addressed by healthcare reform.

REGULATION

Federal, state, and local laws seem designed to make running a small business difficult. Beyond normal regulatory compliance such as tax, pension, wage and hour laws, etc., healthcare has its own set of additional regulations that add complexity. For example, consider some of the laws and complex regulations that apply to even the smallest medical practices:

- OSHA—Occupational Safety and Health Administration
- CLIA—Clinical Laboratory Improvement Amendments
- HIPAA—Health Insurance Portability and Accountability Act
- Medicare (billing, coding, unbundling, supervision requirements, etc.)
- State Medicaid regulations and eligibility requirements
- Third-party payor rules and regulations, which often vary from Medicare
- Self-referral (the Stark Law).

There is no exemption from complying with these and other regulations, and the penalties for not complying are often quite harsh.

REIMBURSEMENT

Starting back in the mid-1980s, commercial insurance companies began developing networks of physicians. They promised reduced paperwork and streamlined payments. No longer would the physician bill the patient who would, in turn, file a claim with the insurance company. Instead, the patient would pay a nominal copayment, and the physician would bill the insurance company and be paid based on a predetermined fee schedule.

The result was that it became easier for insurance companies to market their networks of physicians to employers and sell their insurance products. It sounded like a good deal to the physicians, too—just bill the insurance companies rather than hundreds of individual patients.

Over the years, smaller insurance companies were purchased by larger insurance companies. Recent years have seen mergers of these large insurance companies to the point that many areas of the country are now dominated by a small number of commercial third-party payors. These payors basically control a medical group's commercial patients and wield tremendous market power.

While payments to physician practices were to be based on a negotiated fee schedule, in reality there is very little negotiation. Many physician groups have two options: accept the fee schedule being offered or lose the business.

A few years ago, I worked with a business-astute solo family physician in the Northeast. He knew something was wrong in his practice—he was working harder and making less. He went back and traced actual payments from one of his main commercial payors over the preceding six-year period. He found an average decline of 4.2% per year in payment rates for his major CPT codes and an overall decline during the six-year period of more than 19%!

When he confronted the payor with these data, the company shrugged and told him he was free to terminate the contract. The managed care battle has been fought, and solo and small physician groups lost. They have virtually no leverage in negotiating payment rates. They sold their patients to the insurance companies and got them back at a discount.

As mentioned above, the proliferation of high-deductible plans under the ACA, especially in the individual insurance market but in many company benefit plans too, has greatly increased the complexity and further eroded the ability of a small physician office to bill and collect from patients.

Healthcare for Medicare patients, who usually make up 30% to 60% of a physician practice, is paid for by a system that is in the midst of dramatic change. Medicare implemented a national fee schedule in the 1990s, and for years physician fees were to be automatically adjusted every year based on a statutory formula called the sustainable growth rate (SGR). In simplified terms, the SGR set a global Medicare budget for physician services and divided it by expected utilization based on the Medicare population. The result was the threat of large annual decreases in Medicare's fee schedule. Avoiding the automatic decreases required Congressional action. The result, in some parts of the country, was for physicians to limit access or to stop taking new Medicare patients altogether.

The SGR formula was finally repealed in early 2015 and its replacement sets annual increases in Medicare fees to .5% per year through mid-2019. By 2019, a new system is supposed to be in place to reimburse physicians for Medicare using either a merit payment system or an alternative payment system. Both of these systems will, in different ways, attempt to layer either bonuses or penalties on top of the existing fees for service in an attempt to begin to move away from fee-for-service and base reimbursement, at least in part, on quality measures or sharing of financial risk.

The merit payment system will provide bonuses or penalties starting at 5% in 2019 and increasing to 9% by 2022 for improving quality, resource use, meaningful use of EHRs, and practice improvement activities. Details obviously will have to be worked out.

The alternative payment system requires physicians to join an ACO or be part of an integrated delivery system or a patient-centered medical home. This alternative method, which seems to be where Congress is pushing physicians, will also require performance improvements and financial risk to be defined.

Many regulations will have to be written and the quality metrics will need to be determined and systems in place to measure them. Right now there are more questions than answers, but Medicare clearly is moving toward trying something that will move physician payment away from the current fee-for-service (or some would call it fee-for-volume) system we currently function under.

A majority of commercial payors' fee schedules are based on Medicare's national fee schedule, with commercial rates set as a percentage of Medicare's. Historically, the downward pressure on these rates and now the minimal increases of .5% per year on Medicare fees effective through 2019 could continue to keep commercial reimbursement rates relatively flat as well.

State Medicaid program rates often don't even cover the cost of providing the services and have caused large numbers of physicians to either drop Medicaid altogether or to severely limit the number of these patients they are willing to take on in their practice. The ACA provided some interim relief by requiring that Medicaid payments to primary care physicians equal the Medicare rates during 2013 and 2014 for evaluation and management services and immunizations.

ANCILLARY SERVICES

Ancillary services such as laboratory and diagnostic imaging were once the staple of many successful practices. The ability to generate a profit margin from ancillary services historically represented as much as 20% to 30% of the revenue of a primary care practice—and even more in specialty practices.

Recent years have seen reimbursement changes that make this strategy less lucrative and have even led to the shutdown of these services in some practices.

The Deficit Reduction Act of 2005, which was effective in 2007, reduced Medicare reimbursement on most diagnostic imaging procedures performed in physician offices by 25% to 30%. Commercial payors, whose reimbursement rates often are pegged to a percentage of Medicare, are following these reductions in many parts of the country.

In addition, commercial payors in some parts of the country have been imposing additional requirements on in-office imaging, including the following:

- A requirement that the practice provide a full range of imaging modalities;
- A requirement for a full-time radiologist onsite; and
- Accreditation requirements.

The cost of meeting these requirements makes it difficult, if not impossible, for smaller practices to provide these services.

The ACA included several provisions that resulted in additional payment reductions for many imaging services.

Finally, most commercial payors now use radiology benefit managers and require pre-authorization for many diagnostic tests.

RECRUITMENT AND RETENTION

Recruiting and retaining physicians is increasingly difficult. This problem is driven by three interrelated factors:

1. Physician shortages in many specialties have driven up physician starting salaries. Many physician groups are finding that the starting salary for a newly trained physician is in excess of what senior partners earn. The ACA attempts to address the physician shortage issue, at least in primary care, by providing grants for new or expanded primary care residency programs and tax incentives in underserved areas.

2. Many younger physicians have little interest in the business side of medicine and tend to be more lifestyle- and family-focused than their predecessors. They fear any uncertainty in their incomes—uncertainty tied to the performance of the practice. As a result, they shy away from becoming an owner in the practice. A stable income, regular work hours, and schedule flexibility tend to be their prime concerns, and as a result, many are attracted to hospital employment.

3. 3.   Many areas of the country have become unattractive to both younger and even well-established physicians. Third-party reimbursement rates, poor payor mix, and high malpractice insurance premiums are exacerbating physician access problems in these areas. The higher starting salaries are even harder to support

because the underlying practice economics are worse. The result is physician shortages in these areas.

All of the above factors conspired to make it seem quite compelling to sell to a hospital and become an employee. The hospital seems like a logical shelter from these uncertainties. Hospitals need physicians and have deeper pockets. They may be able to reduce some costs, realize some scale in items such as malpractice insurance, and have more leverage in payor contracting.

ELECTRONIC HEALTH RECORDS

The federal government is committed to moving physician practice into the digital age and is driving the implementation of electronic health records (EHRs) through a series of incentive payments to those who demonstrate "meaningful use" that started in 2011. The incentives turn to penalties for those practices that did not demonstrate meaningful use starting in 2015. The requirements to meet meaningful use can be complex, especially for smaller practices, and the capital cost and lost productivity during the conversion to EHRs is a significant barrier for many physicians.

These initiatives continue. The new Medicare payment systems described above and slated to become effective in 2019 include incentives for meaningful use of EHRs. EHRs will have increased importance under these new payments systems because they are where most of the quality and other performance data that will be used in rewarding or penalizing physicians will come from.

RETIREMENT

Physicians who previously have resisted the option of selling their practice often have a renewed interest as they near retirement. While this interest is often driven by a desire to realize some value for their practice, it is more often driven by the desire to assure some level of continuity of care for their patients as well.

Selling can be a good option here. In fact, in many cases it turns out to be the only option. As discussed above, many younger physicians have little interest in the business side of medicine and are not interested in the financial risks either. Often the options come down to either selling or closing the practice.

Hospitals have a better chance of recruiting a replacement physician because they have deeper pockets—they can afford to pay the recruiting fees and offer market salaries that small independent groups can't. Hospitals also can offer signing bonuses, student loan repayment, moving expense reimbursement, and other benefits that independent groups find difficult to afford.

My advice to physicians nearing retirement and contemplating what to do with their practice is simply this: don't wait too long. Once it is widely known that you have set a retirement date, any value in your practice disappears rapidly. Why? Because once it is known you are going to retire, your patients will be looking for another physician and will become fair game for other physicians, whether they are hospital-employed or independent competitors. In specialty practices, your referral sources will start to migrate as well.

Absent a viable succession plan in your private practice—younger partners and newly recruited associates interested in buying into the practice or buying you out—selling to a hospital may be your only real option.

Rather than just announce your pending retirement in 6–12 months, develop an outline of a transition plan and present it to potential hospital suitors two or three years in advance. A successful transition plan needs to allow plenty of time for execution.

A typical transition plan involves the following:

1. Sale of your practice to the hospital.
2. Joint recruitment by you and the hospital of a physician to replace you upon retirement.
3. Your continuing in practice as a hospital employee while the new physician is recruited and for a period of time afterward during which you gradually reduce your work level and consciously and deliberately transition your patients to the new physician.

As you develop this transition plan, the wild card will be the timing, which needs to be adjusted based on the specific circumstances in your market. For example, if you are in a market where it is difficult to recruit, you should start several years in advance. In other circumstances, perhaps the hospital has recently recruited or even has a currently employed physician working to establish a practice that might be a perfect fit.

One problem that often arises in these situations is the physician who is always "slowing down" or "getting ready to retire" but never seems to reach the point of actually letting go. Physician know thyself in these situations. For a transition plan to work, the commitment to a reasonable timetable will maximize the value of your practice and give you the best chance of success.

SHOULD YOU SELL?

The decision to sell or not sell your practice is a complex one, and it involves much more than financial and security considerations, which are often foremost in the minds of physicians. While these considerations are important—after all, everything has its price and everyone wants security—my experience is that, in the long run, qualitative issues are a much better predictor of satisfaction than quantitative ones.

Though the above factors provide some compelling reasons to sell, it should be noted that many physicians and physician groups both large and small continue not only to survive but thrive in private practice. They are likely to continue to do so in spite of the challenges above. Chapter 10 describes the traits that make these groups successful and provides options and strategies you can adopt to preserve independent private practice if you decide selling your practice is not in your best interest.

Before you go much further, take some time to step back and reflect on:

- Why are you practicing medicine in your current location?
- Why are you in your current practice?
- Why are you in a solo, small-group, large-group, single-specialty or multispecialty group?
- What other types of practice have you tried?

Group practice is like a marriage, and some group practices go bad just like some marriages go bad. Yet usually it isn't the institution of marriage that is the problem but rather the relationship. So why do many physicians have a bad experience in group practice and blame the group structure rather than the individuals?

There are many successful examples of single-specialty and multispecialty groups in most parts of the country. So don't blame your experiences on the institution of group practice without reflecting on what else was at work in a bad situation. Evaluating what you like and dislike about your current structure is a critical first step.

The next questions you have to ask yourself are the following:

- What would change if your practice is sold and you become an employee of a hospital?
- Would you lose some of the things you like, such as autonomy and independence?
- Would the hospital solve some of the things you dislike?

Tread carefully. Just as having children is usually not the best way to resolve marital difficulties, selling your practice may simply move your problems into a different realm. See Checklists 1 and 2 at the end of this chapter to begin your self-evaluation.

I find that many physicians lack the perspective to recognize whether the current situation is objectively good or bad. Sometimes the grass looks greener on the other side. One physician hit the nail on the head when he told me: "I always have to remind myself that it's never as good as it seems on the best days and never as bad as it seems on the worst days. That's how I keep my perspective."

Perspective on your current situation involves multiple components. I worked with an internist a few years ago who was pushing his group practice to sell to the hospital. He had a passionate list of plausible reasons why this was a good move. After spending some time with him and each of his partners individually, I learned that the underlying issue was that this physician didn't get along with his partners, or anyone else for that matter. The question wasn't whether or not they should sell. The question was how being employed by the hospital would solve their intra-group personality problems. They would still be working in the same office and sharing call—and still be financially tied together. What would change?

Many physicians think the decision to sell should be based solely on the monetary offer from the hospital because, after all, "everything has its price." This is a trap, too. As we will see in upcoming chapters, there are many things that are often more important than the monetary terms. Selling a practice is a strategic decision, and it needs to be viewed beyond the realm of short-term financial considerations.

TAKEAWAY POINTS FOR CHAPTER 2

- The trend of physicians selling their practices existed in the market long before the passage of the ACA, which hastened the trend.
- Independent practice faces challenges on many fronts—regulatory, reimbursement, technology, recruitment, and others—and those changes and complexities will continue.
- At this stage, the potential universe of hospital partners has some fairly extensive experience in employing physicians. How are they doing? Are the employed physicians happy with their employment arrangement?
- You must evaluate your true motivation for selling and determine whether the sale will solve any underlying problems.
- Selling your practice is never a panacea—it never solves all your problems and may even introduce some new ones.

Checklist 1: Potential Gains

Use this checklist to evaluate the severity of the problems you hope to solve and the relative importance of the perks you may gain.

Which of these potential "reasons to sell" apply to your situation? Note specifics about how each affects your practice and with what severity.

❏ Regulation and compliance issues _____

_____

❏ Billing and management complexity _____

_____

❏ Restrictions on and declining profitability of ancillary services _____

_____

❏ Lack of leverage in payor contract negotiations _____

_____

❏ Declining reimbursement and reimbursement uncertainty _____

_____

❏ Need to recruit physicians and high starting salaries/physician shortages_____

_____

How important is each potential hospital benefit to you?

❏ Professional practice management_____

_____

❏ Negotiation with third-party payors_____

_____

❏ Attractive benefit packages for staff _____

_____

❑ Potentially lower malpractice insurance rates _____

_____

❑ Retirement plan _____

_____

❑ Health insurance for you and your family _____

_____

❑ Disability insurance _____

_____

❑ Integrated electronic medical records _____

_____

❑ Sophisticated billing and collections systems _____

_____

'

Checklist 2: Evaluating Your Readiness to Sell

Physicians become employees when a hospital owns the practice. Use the questions in this checklist to help you decide if you would be happy in that role.

❏ Are you prepared to turn over at least some control of your work schedule to fit in with the hospital's policies?

❏ Do you currently have scheduling flexibility (like leaving early on Fridays) that may not fit in with corporate expectations?

❏ Would you look forward to adopting new ways to make your practice more efficient? Or does the thought of using a new practice management system or EHR system make your head ache?

❏ Do you want to learn to work in a way that pulls in more money? Or would you resent a hospital "suit" giving you guidelines for increasing the number of patients you see?

❏ Are you ready and willing to trade away any upside potential for protection from downside risk?

❏ Do you hope to rid yourself of personnel decisions? Or does giving up some control of your staff feel too risky?

❏ What was your relationship with or attitude toward hospital management when you were in your residency program?

❏ Do you know and respect the leadership of local hospitals?

❏ Have you talked with other physicians who have sold their practices? Do you think their good and bad experiences would apply to your situation? How?

CHAPTER 3

Preparing Your Practice for Sale

Charming home in established neighborhood. In original condition.
Needs TLC.   REAL ESTATE ADVERTISEMENT

You probably wouldn't put a "For Sale" sign in your front lawn without some preparation, and the same applies to putting your practice on the market. The biggest mistake physicians make in selling is that they jump in without adequate preparation. Planning ahead to make your business as attractive and valuable as possible is critical. Selling a practice, like selling a house, means that taking the time to prepare it for sale can pay off handsomely.

First, step back and look at the real estate equivalent of curb appeal. How will your practice look to a potential purchaser? I have a friend who claims that all antiques become antiques only after passing through the phase where they are a "piece of junk." I see many practices with waiting rooms where the furniture and décor is in this near-antique stage.

Furniture isn't the only thing that impacts perception. Is the paint peeling off the door? Is the carpet worn and stained? Is your signage faded and dated? While these things may not directly impact the financial valuation of your practice, they will impact the *perception* of your practice to a potential purchaser, and perception often becomes reality.

Most hospitals are very image-conscious. They invest heavily in their main entrances, waiting rooms, landscaping, and even color selection in order to project a calming yet professional image. What image do they have of you and your practice?

I'm not suggesting the Taj Mahal either. I worked with one solo physician whose wife spent $50,000 decorating the waiting room. A modern and tasteful image is what you are looking for.

When dressing up your practice for sale, don't fall into the trap of thinking you'll somehow be more attractive to a hospital if you invest in state-of-the-art technology. Technology investments have some of the shortest useful lives of any assets you will purchase. A five-year-old computer is ancient, and software depreciates at a rapid rate.

Don't invest in an expensive EHR system or new practice management software if you are planning to sell. Transitioning to a new EHR system takes valuable time and cuts into productivity, at least initially. Changing your billing system always results in short-term cash flow reductions. As a hospital administrator I worked with last year quipped, "There are no good computer conversions, only varying degrees of bad."

The hospital you affiliate with may not use your hardware and software anyway, so your investment will have minimal value to them, and you will likely have another learning curve post-acquisition.

If you do purchase other major equipment within a year or two of selling, be sure to keep good records to justify the value, but don't hold your breath. Computer hardware has minimal resale value in today's market and unless it is compatible with the hospital's system, they may even decline to purchase it. Software likewise often has little, if any, value and in many cases is licensed and cannot readily be sold or transferred. Make sure these items are taken into account when your practice is being priced.

FINANCIAL PERFORMANCE

Instead of the purchases described above, concentrate on achieving positive revenue trends and generating above-average income. Your financial performance is the most important aspect of your income post-sale, and maybe even the hospital's level of interest. Many hospitals will shy away from a practice with subpar finances or one viewed as faltering and in need of a turnaround. Financial performance can be broken down into three main components: physician income, revenue, and overhead. Let's examine each of these in more detail.

PHYSICIAN INCOME

Your income is a driving factor behind the value of your practice and is a key aspect of your preparation to sell. The compensation package you are offered by the hospital will likely be based on your current income. The hospital's ability to successfully operate your practice and manage its finances will also be driven by your income expectations.

Before you place your practice on the market—before you approach a hospital or share any financial data—you need to know how your income compares with your peers and why.

Quantifying physician income can be a bit nebulous in smaller practices. Every dollar collected that is not spent on overhead is available for physician income, but that is not necessarily what shows up on a physician's W-2 form.

Many practices have generous physician-owner benefits such as health, life, and disability insurance, as well as retirement plan contributions. High levels of physician discretionary expenses such as auto expenses, meals, travel and entertainment, and continuing education also can lead to an understatement of the true earning ability of a practice.

Physician income is usually "normalized" to adjust for varying levels of these nonstandard physician benefits and other discretionary expenses so it more accurately reflects physician income. The valuation firm the hospital engages (Chapter 5) will examine and adjust for these expenses. You may need to work with your CPA or practice consultant to obtain a more accurate estimate of your earning ability. For a quick estimate, simply add any physician expenses that you feel may be a bit extravagant to your W-2 income.

Once your true earnings are estimated, compare that income with that of your peers. The Medical Group Management Association (MGMA; www.mgma.com) publishes annual surveys of physician income by specialty, group size, geographic location, and years in practice. The American Medical Group Association (AMGA; www.amga.org) is another resource.

A Word About Surveys

While the MGMA and AMGA surveys are comprehensive and an excellent resource, other resources are available as well. These surveys include substantial data and a majority of hospitals and their consultants use them extensively on a daily basis.

It is important to apply a degree of skepticism of these surveys and this has become increasingly true as more and more physicians have become employees of hospitals. There are several obvious biases in the survey data. Some of this bias is environmental—that is, the bias is a byproduct of the marketplace and demographics of the survey respondents. Some of the bias is what I call self-fulfilling, caused by continual misuse of the survey data year over year by hospitals and practice management professionals. Both physicians and hospitals should be aware of the following biases and recognize the limitations of the survey data:

Respondent Bias

The survey data are solely a reflection of the physician practices that respond. Respondents typically receive a complimentary copy of the final survey document but are otherwise not compensated for completing the survey, which is a complex and time-consuming task.

Small private practices generally do not have the resources or even the ability to compile the data necessary to respond and, as a result, go virtually unrepresented in the survey data. This leaves survey responses dominated by large medical groups and increasingly by those owned by hospital systems. Many of the surveys no longer have respondents from a sufficient number of physician-owned practices to permit publishing separate survey data for independent physicians.

This respondent bias tends to overstate physician compensation and understate physician productivity. The huge losses being subsidized by hospitals employing physicians shown in Chapter 1 mean that physician compensation being reported by these hospitals reflect a false economic reality. In private practice, physician compensation is generally what is left after paying overhead, which is a true reflection of the economic earnings of that physician. The salary survey data that are increasingly dominated by hospital-employed physicians are not a true reflection of what a physician can earn in private practice.

Conversely, productivity, which is usually defined in terms of work relative value units (wRVUs), discussed further below, generally declines for hospital-employed physicians. These declines, when reported on the surveys, drive down the reported levels of physician productivity. Since the survey responses are increasingly weighted toward hospital-employed physicians, the productivity of small practices, largely unrepresented in the survey data, tends to be higher than what is reported in the surveys.

Self-fulfilling Bias

Self-fulfilling bias is introduced and exacerbated by the continual misuse of the survey data year over year. The compensation reported in the surveys generally includes *all* physician compensation. Yet many hospitals, compensation appraisers, consultants, other advisors, and even physicians use the reported compensation as a basis for establishing clinical compensation. Additional compensation for nonproductivity compensation such as "quality," administrative compensation, call coverage, and other stipends, are added on top.

In subsequent years, this additional compensation is added to the clinical compensation and reported in the surveys, which results in an artificial increase in reported compensation and then, the next year, the self-perpetuating cycle begins again.

Takeaway Points on Surveys

My company looks at the performance of dozens of independent physician practices each year and virtually all of them have physician incomes below and physician productivity above what is being reported in the survey data.

Hospitals' reliance on the survey data is becoming almost universal. Several years ago it was rare that a hospital would even have access to the survey data and now virtually all hospitals purchase the surveys.

It is ironic that the increased reliance on the survey data—viewed by many hospital systems as a "bible"—comes at a time when, for the reasons stated above, the survey data itself are not an accurate reflection of the economic performance of a physician-owned private practice.

Both hospital employees and physicians and physician practice managers should be aware of these issues with the survey data. It is not "gospel," and care should be taken in their use, or in many cases, misuse.

Your CPA or practice consultant should have access to this information and can help you complete the comparisons and sift through the issues discussed in this chapter.

REVENUE

A vast majority of practices I have worked with over the past 25 years that have below-average physician incomes have revenue issues. Ideally you want to show the hospital that your revenue is average or above for your specialty and that your revenue is growing each year. This tells the hospital that your practice is thriving, which will make your practice more attractive and support a higher valuation. Declining revenue trends, even by only 1% or 2% per year, can be construed as a declining practice.

Compare your revenue with the MGMA or other surveys. Revenue does vary, often dramatically, by geographic region, so make sure your comparison is specific to your location. If your revenue is lower than that of your peers, you will need to drill down to determine why. Revenue is composed of several components that will need to be examined individually.

Productivity includes the number of patients you see, the number of procedures you perform, and the CPT codes you apply to those patient visits and procedures. This is the component doctors can most easily impact.

The MGMA surveys publish data on the number of patient encounters. Compare the encounter data of your practice with the survey results to determine what part your personal productivity plays in your revenue.

Productivity can be below average for many reasons. You may need to examine your work schedule, time off, scheduling templates, work habits, and other factors. A degree of self-assessment may be required. Taking the time to understand your productivity now will also be helpful when it comes to negotiating with the hospital later (Chapter 8). Most hospitals will seek to base your post-sale bonus or even your base salary on your ability to maintain or attain a specified level of production.

Coding also affects revenue. Many physicians have the propensity to under-code, often because they fear payor chart audits. Taking the time to learn and follow proper coding and documentation procedures can enhance your revenue without significant additional work—better documentation of work you are already doing can result in increases in revenue.

Some physicians are on the opposite end of this spectrum—they tend to be too aggressive in coding. This has the opposite effect as it tends to overstate revenue. Many hospitals will review your coding and documentation for compliance before the sale and monitor it for compliance post-sale. If you have a tendency to be aggressive in coding, you may find your productivity declines after the sale.

Work relative value units (wRVUs) are the best way to measure and benchmark productivity because they take into account both of the above factors—work effort and coding. wRVUs are the underpinning of most physician reimbursement, although many physicians either don't know what they are or view them with a level of distrust. RVUs are part of the resource-based relative value scale (RBRVS) that transitioned to a standardized Medicare physician payment method back 1992.

RVUs are assigned to each procedure performed by healthcare providers. As the name implies, wRVUs measure *work* effort of one procedure relative to another. Specifically, wRVUs take into account the following:

- Physician time required to perform the service;
- Technical skill and physical effort;
- Mental effort and judgment; and
- Psychological stress associated with physician's concern about the risk to the patient.

Perhaps the easiest way for physicians to think of wRVUs is to think of one of the most commonly used CPT codes 99213—Office/outpatient visit, established patient level 3—as 1 wRVU (actually, it is .97 wRVU). Contrast that with CPT code 99214—Office/outpatient visit, established patient level 4—at 1.5 wRVUs, and you begin to understand how it works.

Since the government is involved, naturally it isn't as simple as it sounds. For one thing, wRVU values can and do change periodically, and such changes are generally required to be revenue neutral to Medicare. So if one CPT code's wRVU value goes up others will go down.

There are two other types of RVUs: practice expense (PE) and malpractice (MP). These two types are adjusted for geographic cost factors to reflect local or regional variances in operating expenses and the risk of malpractice claims inherent in individual CPT codes.

The total of these three RVUs (work, PE, and MP) are finally multiplied by a national conversion factor to arrive at the allowable payment amount for the Medicare physician fee schedule.

The beauty of wRVUs is that they are universal across all specialties and geographic regions. So if you can determine your wRVUs, which as noted above inherently take into account both your volume of work effort and your coding, it becomes easy to compare your productivity with that of other physicians in your specialty on a national basis.

How do you determine your wRVUs? wRVU values for each CPT code are published at least annually as part of the Medicare Physician Fee Schedule and are available at the Centers for Medicare & Medicaid Services (CMS) Web site at www.cms.gov/physicianfeesched/pfsrvf/list.asp as well as at many other Internet sites. Care must be taken if you or your office manager undertake this effort manually, however, as raw wRVUs often need to be adjusted based on use of CPT code modifiers. Your practice consultant may need to help you with these adjustments.

Many newer practice management software packages also provide wRVU data, although I urge caution here, too. As noted above, wRVU values can and do change so you want to be sure your software provider has updated the values in your system. Outdated wRVU values in practice billing systems, in my experience, are the rule rather than the exception.

There are many other resources that can cost effectively determine your wRVUs. One resource I like is the InfoDive® tool offered by Trellis Healthcare (www.trellishc.com).

There are other pitfalls in ensuring that you have accurate wRVU data. For example, if your practice uses midlevel providers such as physician assistants or nurse practitioners, you want to make sure you are not counting their wRVUs for services billed under your name ("incident-to") as part of your productivity.

Once you have accurate wRVU data, a whole world of accurate benchmarking opens to you. The MGMA and AMGA surveys contain extensive wRVU data by specialty and geographic region. Try comparing yourself in the following areas, but remember the discussion of survey data, above: wRVU data in the surveys tend to be understated because of the biases noted.

1. Compare your productivity in terms of wRVUs to others in your specialty by percentile.
2. Divide your collections by your wRVUs and compare your collections per wRVU with that of your peers and colleagues around the country. Remember, though, that revenue per wRVU will also reflect varying payment rates across geographic locations because payments include those PE and MP RVUs discussed above. So, for example, you would expect practices in areas with a higher cost of living, such as New York City/Northern New Jersey, to have higher collections per wRVU than rural areas.
3. Divide your income by your wRVUs and compare your income per wRVU with that of your peers around the country (although the potential distortion mentioned above on cost of living applies here as well).

The wRVU Benchmarking Worksheet at the end of this chapter can aid you in making these calculations.

Taking the time to obtain accurate historical wRVUs has another very important benefit—it will ensure you are prepared when it comes time to sit down and discuss compensation with the hospital. As discussed in detail in Chapter 6, hospital compensation plans have evolved in the past few years to almost universally rely on wRVUs. You will find it very beneficial to have your own data to compare to the hospital's analysis, and it will make it much easier to assess how your wRVUs fit into the hospital's compensation model and the impact on your personal income.

Billing and collections is another revenue component. If your revenue is below the median for your specialty but your wRVUs are in line, this is the next area to examine.

The most common problems in billing and collections are in the failure to collect copayments. Copayments increasingly represent a huge percentage of what most physicians are paid for an office visit. They should be collected before the patient is seen. Billing patients for copayments is inefficient and may even violate the terms of your payor contracts.

Another area you should review is your financial policies. Many practices continue to provide care to patients who have significant, old outstanding balances. While there are ethical concerns that need to be considered, ignoring these balances and continuing to provide care sends the wrong message. You may decide to provide some free care, but that is different than allowing your system to accumulate bad debt that you will never collect. You may want to look at options such as payment plans rather than writing off outstanding balances.

Here are some simple additional steps you can take to uncover red flags in your billing department:

1. Take a look at your total monthly collection trend or simply the receipts being deposited in your bank account monthly for the past two years. If your work schedule and patient volumes have been steady, your receipts should be, too. Most practices will have some variance seasonally, so looking at a three- or six-month rolling average can even out short-term fluctuations. Declining collection trends warrant further investigation.

2. Review your gross collection percentage trend (collections divided by gross charges) over the past few years. A declining gross collection percentage, in the absence of significant increases in your standard fee schedule, is an indication of billing problems or declining reimbursement rates.

3. Review your accounts receivable aging trend. An accounts receivable aging is a listing of total balances outstanding by age, such as 0 to 30 days, 30 to 60 days, 60 to 90 days, etc. A trend of increasing balances in the 60- to 90-day and over-90-day categories means collections are falling behind. Balances over 90 days are generally not collectible.

Be wary of accounts receivable aging reports that look too perfect. Sometimes billing personnel or even practice managers will write off old balances to make the aging reports look good.

As noted above, *reimbursement* rates for both commercial payors and Medicare/Medicaid vary widely by geographic area. As discussed in Chapter 2, most small practices have little ability to negotiate with commercial payors. If your patient-encounter volumes meet or exceed national standards, your coding is correct, and there are no obvious problems in your billing department, it may be that your lower revenue is simply a reflection of low reimbursement. I urge caution here. Poor reimbursement is a common excuse used to mask poor billing and collections.

The sheer amount of billing data in a practice can make any review of reimbursement rates seem overwhelming. Think of it as detective work, and don't let it become daunting. Consider that in most practices, the top 20 CPT codes and three or four payors usually account for 80% to 90% of revenue.

Obtain and periodically review explanations of benefits (EOBs) from your top one or two payors, or have your office manager do so. Pay attention to what you are being paid for your most common CPT codes. Compare these rates to what they were one and two years ago.

This doesn't have to be a major project. Ask to see a random EOB from one of your major commercial payors from a random month for each of the past three years. You will quickly see whether reimbursement rates are declining and what impact that is having on your revenue.

The Reimbursement Worksheet at the end of this chapter will help in this analysis.

OVERHEAD AND OVERHEAD PERCENTAGE

If you have followed the above examination of revenue, you should have a pretty good idea of how your revenue compares with that of your peers and how it impacts your income. Now it is finally time to look at overhead. Most physicians want to look at overhead first, and while some practices do have bloated overhead, this is the exception rather than the rule.

You will need to determine your overhead percentage (overhead divided by revenue) and compare that with the MGMA survey results. To do so, you will need to determine your "operating overhead."

Operating overhead doesn't include the salary and benefit costs of you or any other physician or midlevel provider in your practice. Nor does operating overhead include the physician discretionary expenses discussed above. The Income/Overhead Percentage Worksheet at the end of this chapter will help you determine your operating overhead to facilitate this comparison.

Unfortunately, here too, there are problems with the survey data. In many cases there are insufficient response rates from physician-owned practices to allow publication of meaningful cost survey data, and comparing the operating costs of a hospital-owned practice to a physician-owned practice can be like comparing apples with watermelons.

Regardless what this comparison says, it is important to recognize that overhead percentage is the most misused statistic in medical practice management. A high overhead percentage compared with the MGMA survey results does not necessarily mean your overhead is too high.

Overhead percentage is the ratio of overhead to revenue. So revenue is a part of the equation as well. If you've completed the above analysis of your revenue and determined that your revenue is below average, you should already know that your overhead percentage is overstated. Your overhead percentage will magically go down when your revenue goes up. So don't jump to conclusions without looking objectively at both sides of the equation.

If your revenue is on par with national standards, then a high overhead percentage may indeed mean your overhead really is high. If this is the case, once again, you have to drill down.

In most practices, the largest component of overhead is in salaries and benefits. Take a look at your staffing levels per physician and compare them with MGMA data. Review your salary levels and employee benefits. Many practices with low staff turnover find themselves with salary levels that are above prevailing market rates and find their benefits more generous than other practices in the area.

Take a look at what you're spending for drugs and supplies. A practice attitude that "company money" can be spent frivolously dramatically increases overhead.

TAKING ACTION

If you've found problems with your income, revenue, or overhead, you should begin to take corrective action before you go any further in pursuing the sale of your practice. As noted above, many hospitals aren't interested in purchasing practices in need of a major turnaround, and selling at this point will likely result in a substandard financial arrangement for you, too. It is also unlikely that the sale of your practice will resolve many of the problems you have uncovered.

Your goal at this point should be to take the appropriate action to make your practice a stellar performer. This may require you to spend more time on business issues than you'd like, and it may require changes in policies, services, and personnel.

Preparing your practice for sale also means you need to step back and think in a broader strategic sense. There's an old adage that holds: "If you keep doing what you're doing, you'll keep getting what you're getting."

Strategically consider your practice's market position. Who is your competition, and what are they doing? What can you do to improve your market share, volumes, visibility, and standing in the community? These are things that most small practices spend too little time thinking about because the physicians are too busy seeing patients.

Don't overlook potential sources of revenue because of the overhead cost. For example, mid-level provider salaries are on the rise as demand for those services increases, but these professionals nationally generate a gross profit margin (that is, direct incremental revenue in excess of direct cost) equal to or in excess of the profit margin of a physician. Many practices still resist the opportunity to enhance their incomes using midlevel providers out of fear that their overhead will go up.

Midlevel providers offer practices a chance to increase provider capacity and market share without a huge long-term investment, and the return on that investment can be realized in 6 to 12 months. They don't expect to become partners in the practice, and their gross profit trickles down to bolster physician income and vastly enhance the value of the practice to a potential hospital purchaser.

If you already employ midlevel providers, look for ways to increase their productivity through better utilization. Consider extended office hours. Consider establishing disease management clinics staffed primarily by midlevel providers, for example, in diabetes care or management of lipids.

Make sure your practice is providing the full range of ancillary services for your specialty. I still see internal medicine groups without basic lab facilities and cardiology groups without nuclear capabilities. These services add significantly to the bottom line that is so important to maximizing your value with a hospital.

Stepping back and taking the time to understand your practice's performance will be invaluable whether you ultimately sell or not.

HOSPITAL PERSPECTIVE

Hospitals, especially those with experience in acquiring and employing physicians, are going to be more interested in well-run, financially growing practices. Hospitals with experience and expertise in managing physician practices will accept the challenges needed to turn around below-average practices, but high-performing practices will be worth more and provide less acquisition risk to the hospital.

Despite what most physicians think, hospitals are more than willing to pay top dollar for well-run practices and top salaries to top-earning physicians because these practices and physicians help them meet their business goals faster and with less effort.

TAKEAWAY POINTS FOR CHAPTER 3

1. The biggest mistake physicians make in selling is that they jump in without adequate preparation. Planning ahead to make your business as attractive and valuable as possible is a critical first step.
2. You will need to step back and look at the real estate equivalent of curb appeal.
3. Your practice won't be more attractive to a hospital suitor if you invest in state-of-the-art technology.
4. Your financial performance is the most important aspect of selling your practice. It will drive the value of your practice, your income post-sale, and maybe even the hospital's level of interest.

5. Your income is a driving factor behind the value of your practice and is a key aspect of your preparation to sell.

6. If your income is significantly below the MGMA median for your specialty in your geographic location, you need to find out why, but be cautious in over-relying on the survey data because of the biases discussed in this chapter.

7. A vast majority of practices I have worked with over the past 20 years that have below-average physician incomes are in that situation as a result of revenue issues.

8. Revenue trends declining even by only 1% or 2% per year can be construed as a declining practice.

9. Revenue is made up of several components, and if your revenue is below average, these should be examined individually: productivity, coding, billing and collections, and reimbursement rates.

10. You need to learn about and understand wRVUs, as they are the best way to benchmark your productivity, coding, revenue, and income to others in your specialty.

11. While some practices do have bloated overhead, this is the exception rather than the rule.

12. Overhead percentage is the most misused statistic in medical practice management. A high overhead percentage does not necessarily mean your overhead is too high. Your overhead percentage will magically go down when your revenue goes up.

13. If you've found problems with your income, revenue, or overhead, you need to take corrective action before you go any further in pursuing the sale of your practice.

14. Preparing your practice for sale also means you need to step back and think in a broader strategic sense, perhaps looking for additional revenue streams. Stepping back and taking the time to understand your practice's performance will be invaluable whether you sell or not.

Checklist: How Pretty Is Your Practice?

Use this checklist to rate the curb appeal and staging of your practice, because these elements affect the potential purchaser's perception of your practice even if they don't affect the financial valuation. (This also affects patients' and potential patients' perceptions, too, of course.)

Physical Component	Rating (Good, Fair, Bad)	Notes for Improvement (If Needed)
Building exterior		
Building interior hallway and front door		
Condition of waiting room furniture: Is it welcoming and tidy?		
Condition of flooring?		
Reception desk: Is it easily identified and approachable by patients? Is the area relatively clutter-free?		
Exam rooms: Attractive and adequately equipped?		
Physician offices: Do they reflect a well-managed practice?		
Equipment: Does it appear well-maintained even if older?		

Income/Overhead Percentage Worksheet

Income/Overhead Percentage Worksheet	
A. Practice Revenue	
B. Physician and Provider Salaries, Benefits and Discretionary Expenses	
Physician owner salary or net income	
+ Associate physician salaries	
+ Mid-level provider salaries	
+ Provider payroll taxes	
+ Provider health, life, and disability insurance benefits	
+ Provider pension and profit sharing contributions	
+ Auto expense	
+ Continuing education	
+ Travel expense	
+ Meals and entertainment	
+ Other provider discretionary expenses	
B. Total Physician Provider Salaries and Benefits	
C. (A − B) = True Practice Overhead	
D. (C ÷ A) = True Practice Overhead Percentage	
E. Benchmark Overhead Percentage	

Reimbursement Worksheet

Complete for your top 20 CPT codes for Medicare and your top two to four payors. Actual payments should include copays.

CPT® Code	Medicare Allowable Fee	Actual Payment from _____ (payor name)	_____ (payor name) Payment Percent of Medicare

wRVU Benchmarking Worksheet

	Physician Name _____	**Approximate Survey Percentile**
wRVUs		
Revenue		
Revenue per wRVU		
Physician Income		
Physician Income per wRVU		

CHAPTER 4

Choosing the Right Hospital Partner

In choosing a partner, always pick the optimist.
TONY LEMA

C hoosing the right hospital partner is key to a long-term successful relationship. All hospitals are not created equal when it comes to being physician-friendly and having a commitment to long-term success with practice
acquisition and physician employment strategy. Hospitals that lack experience should
be looked at with a healthy degree of skepticism.

HISTORICAL BACKGROUND

As noted in Chapter 1, in the mid- to late-2000s hospitals were purchasing physician
practices at a rate not seen since the 1990s, and the action was widespread. Back then,
many thought this trend would be a repeat of the 1990s. A short history lesson is in
order. The 1990s saw a feeding frenzy of hospitals snapping up physician practices.
Bidding wars erupted in many areas of the country, and prices were driven up as
a result. This trend toward integration was driven by two main factors: efforts at
healthcare reform legislation and physician practice management companies.

The healthcare reform proposed by the Clinton administration had its underpinning in capitation and large integrated networks. Hospitals' acquisition of practices
was initially driven by their desire to develop an adequate physician network.

Practice management companies were pioneered by Nashville-based PhyCor.
Literally dozens of copycats followed, fueled by Wall Street venture capital and
public stock offerings. The model was really quite simple: the practice management
company would offer the physicians a payment for their practice—usually in stock
or a combination of stock and cash up front—in exchange for a long-term (30- to
40-year) management contract. The companies' entry into the physician acquisition
market resulted in competition with hospitals, and that further drove up prices.

Practice management companies didn't do a very good job of managing practices. Wall Street demanded growth to keep the companies' stock prices up, and that growth was easier to fuel by acquiring more and larger practices than by actually managing those they had already acquired. The practices they had purchased became disenchanted by the high management fees and perceived lack of management and, in the end, sought termination of the management agreements. The growth needed to produce higher stock prices was unsustainable, and the whole practice management company industry came crashing down and virtually disappeared from the scene in a very short period of time.

Hospitals, for the most part, did an even worse job of managing physician practices. Hampered by long-term salary guarantees demanded by physicians, coupled with a lack of physician productivity standards, productivity fell by 20% to 25%.

Hospitals also often layered-on corporate overhead, so their promises of reducing overhead often resulted in permanent increases instead. Many hospitals didn't invest in experienced physician practice professionals, physician billing systems, and financial controls. Many of the hospitals that did hire professionals dedicated those professionals to focusing on acquiring more practices.

When the losses mounted, hospitals often responded by cutting staff in the practices, which further hampered efforts to stimulate productivity. Within a year or two, hospitals were losing an average of $100,000 per physician annually, and that didn't include the huge upfront investments they had made in acquiring practices. The acquisition binge became a divestiture binge. An implosion similar to that of the practice management companies took place. Long-time CEOs were dismissed, many hospitals had their debt ratings lowered, and some hospitals even had to be sold as a result of the huge losses sustained.

Physicians found themselves facing the reality that they had been overpaid and that their future incomes were going to be less. Many physicians' incomes never approached the levels they had under the cushy deals with hospitals.

When the current cycle of acquisition and employment of physician practices started again in the mid- to late-2000s, many physicians thought it was simply a repeat of those heady days of the 1990s. Initially it most assuredly was not. It initially seemed that the lessons from that debacle had been learned and that this time, hospitals were approaching the business of acquiring and managing physician practices much differently. For a while, the hospital industry was able to avoid big buyouts and long-term salary guarantees.

As noted earlier, the passage of the ACA in March 2010 only hastened the trend of physician practice sales to hospitals—a trend that was present for several years before passage of health reform. There are some similarities to the 1990s, however.

The underpinning of health reform this time around isn't capitation but new payment models that have eerily similar characteristics. Bundled payments, coordination or integration of care, quality initiatives, ACOs, and the patient-centered medical home (PCMH) are recurring themes of reform. Many believe they will ultimately lead to payment mechanisms that are not based on volume but on coordination of care, quality, and outcomes. There are multiple pilot projects already underway in these areas, and it may be increasingly difficult for small independent practices to "play" under these new payment mechanisms without being part of a larger organization, although the jury is still out. The other similarity that has emerged as the ACA has been implemented is the previous restraint being exercised by hospitals in their physician acquisition and compensation models has been thrown by the wayside in many markets.

There are many reasons for this, and the primary one is simply supply and demand: as the supply of available independent groups has dwindled through acquisition and employment, the price for those remaining has increased. This is especially true with large single- and multispecialty groups that became the remaining "prizes" in certain markets, and bidding wars, which were largely unseen before the ACA, have erupted in some markets, driving acquisition prices and compensation offers to what I believe are unsustainable levels.

HOSPITAL MOTIVATIONS

Hospitals, of course, aren't purchasing practices for altruistic reasons. Hospitals need physicians to maintain and grow market share, support service lines, and show third-party payors they have an extensive network of providers to serve the payors' patient base. They need critical mass to "play" in the expected future bundled payment modes, ACOs, PCMHs, and other initiatives.

In smaller, nonurban markets, hospitals can substantially grow market share by stopping out-migration of patients to larger urban hospitals by offering an expanded range of specialty services. Attracting specialty physicians to provide those services requires a robust primary care base to support those specialties, as well as hospital services such as diagnostic testing and surgery.

Hospitals in urban areas with intense competition seek to make inroads into the competition's market share by expanding both their primary care and specialty physi-

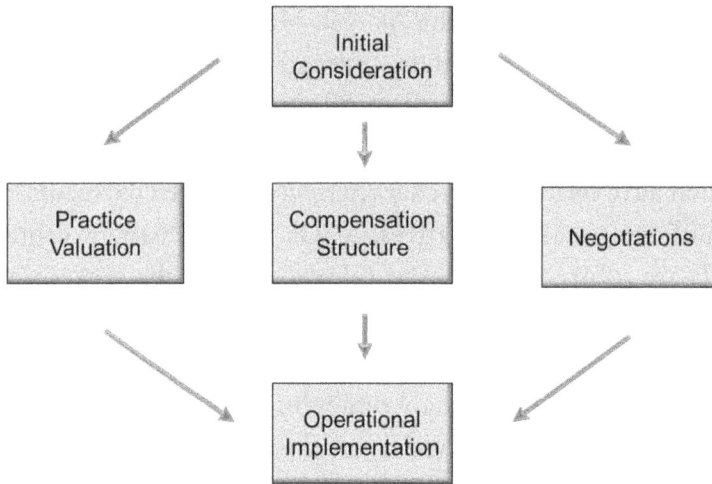

FIGURE 4-1. Hospital Acquisition Process

cian base. They can do this by recruiting new physicians to the community or attracting physicians from competing hospitals with offers of employment and security.

HOSPITAL ACQUISITION PROCESS

The basic process you and the hospital will go through in acquiring your practice is illustrated in Figure 4-1.

The basic steps include completing a valuation and related due diligence on your practice, and proposing a practice acquisition price and compensation structure. Negotiations and legal agreements with you and your advisors follow, detailing the structure of the transactions. As in selling a house, these negotiations lead to a formal closing followed by a specific date when you commence practice as an employee of the hospital. All of these steps are discussed in detail in the following chapters.

HOSPITAL VIABILITY

At this initial stage, your goal should be to take an objective view of the hospital(s) you may be interested in joining. If a hospital approaches you, you should use this chapter to gain an understanding of its models, plans, and strategies for practice acquisition. You should also understand where the hospital is in the cycle of physician employment discussed in Chapter 1.

The first thing to do is examine the business viability of the hospital you are considering. The hospital industry certainly didn't emerge unscathed by the ACA. The promise of a decline in the uninsured was counterbalanced by the emergence of high-deductible health insurance plans. Ask for current financial statements, and, if you don't understand them, work with your accountant to decipher the institution's financial picture. Pay particular attention to volume and cost trends.

If the hospital is independent, consider the likelihood of it being acquired or merging in the foreseeable future. Many hospitals operate on small margins, and while many still have deep pockets, the trend is toward being part of larger systems and this trend has accelerated post-ACA, as many smaller hospitals have come to believe they need to be part of a much larger system to "play" in the "new world" of accountable care and population health management.

Hospitals that are part of larger systems are much more likely to invest in and maintain the practice management infrastructure necessary for successful practice management. The most important component of practice management infrastructure is personnel. Larger hospital systems are better at recruiting and retaining top-level practice management professionals and, more importantly, giving them the autonomy to manage the practices.

Investment in technology—for things such as an EHR system and state-of-the art practice management and billing systems—are critical, too. But remember, especially when dealing with hospitals inexperienced in acquiring physician practices, it is easy to throw money at technology. It is much more difficult to retain the professional management staff necessary to make that technology work.

QUESTIONS TO ASK

(Questions are repeated as a checklist at the end of this chapter.)

While hospitals learned a lot from employing physicians in the 1990s, some didn't embody the lessons. Running a hospital department is different than running a physician practice. Make sure the hospital you choose has committed or is willing to commit to the necessary investment in physician practice management infrastructure and expertise.

The hospital should take a healthy, proactive approach to practice acquisition. Ask about its reasons for buying practices. The answers you are looking for include the following:

- Long-term strategy to grow or maintain market share;
- Response to competitive threats;
- Ability to better serve patients;

- Strategic preparation for new payment and integrated delivery models;
- Increased leverage in negotiation with third-party payors; and
- Desire to help medical staff members survive and thrive.
- Answers that should send up red flags might include the following:
- Competitors buying practices; and
- Ability to cut your overhead.

Ask a lot of questions about the hospital's practice management commitment, and be leery if you don't get specific answers:

1. How many physicians does the hospital currently employ?
2. How many practices does it plan to acquire?
3. Have they had any physicians leave hospital employment? Who? How many? Why?
4. What practice management expertise does the hospital currently have?
5. What practice management positions does the hospital anticipate adding in the future and/or what kind of background is it looking for to fill those positions?
6. How does it do, or plan to do, billing?
7. Does the hospital use provider-based, charging a separate facility fee to patients for office visits?
8. Will billing be a centralized function, or will each practice keep its existing billing system?
9. Does it currently use or have plans for an EHR system?
10. Who will actually negotiate managed care contracts?
11. What is the hospital's business plan for practice acquisition and management?
12. How does my practice fit into that plan?

Talk to those physicians who have already gone through the acquisition process and ask:

1. How was it handled?
2. Are they happy?
3. Has the hospital been willing to work with them to resolve problems and issues?
4. Are they aware of unhappy physicians leaving hospital employment?

Don't be afraid to ask questions specific to your situation:

1. Will you have a say in the hiring and termination of staff?
2. How will staff work rules be enforced?
3. Will you have input into staff evaluations, raises, and bonuses?
4. Can your office be moved or consolidated with another office without your approval?

While some details will have to be worked out in the future, and things will evolve as the number of physicians the hospital employs grows, getting "We'll figure that out later" as the answer to most of your questions should be a red flag as to how well the hospital has thought through its strategy.

Consider your past relationship with the hospital:

1. Is the hospital part of a larger system that has the financial resources necessary to ensure long-term stability?
2. Is administration stable and trusted or is there a lot of turnover?
3. Do you look up to members of the management team as good leaders and role models?
4. Who will be your liaison?
5. Are the individuals in charge experienced and competent, and are they honest and forthright in their business dealings?

Another consideration is how you would feel about answering to hospital administration. If you have had conflicts with administration in the past, you'll have to decide if you can put those behind you and work in close partnership moving forward.

Remember, too, that even if you have a rosy relationship with the hospital CEO and others, turnover at the executive level in hospitals tends to be fairly active. There is no guarantee that the people you deal with today will be in their positions a few years from now. Given that possibility, make sure all points of your agreement are in writing. What he or she said way back when matters little if a whole new team takes over the executive suite.

Ask yourself what the hospital has to offer that will improve the quality of your professional and/or personal life. Then consider if what it is offering is enough for you to give up your autonomy. An attractive buyout price, a solid compensation and benefits package, fewer administrative hassles, and more time for direct patient care might align quite well with your long-term career values and goals.

Understanding a hospital's motivation and strategy, along with its commitment to practice management infrastructure and foresight in evolving as new payment models emerge, is key in choosing the right hospital partner. It is not the hospital with the best offer that is likely to sustain you should you decide to sell—rather, it is the hospital with the commitment to practice management infrastructure, a solid business plan, and the successful execution of that plan.

TAKEAWAY POINTS FOR CHAPTER 4

1. Choosing the right hospital partner is key to a long-term successful relationship.
2. All hospitals are not created equal when it comes to being physician-friendly and having the commitment to a long-term strategy for successful practice acquisition and physician employment.
3. Hospitals that lack experience should be looked at with a healthy degree of skepticism.
4. While hospitals are purchasing physician practices at a rate not seen since the 1990s, try to understand where the hospital is in the cycle of physician employment using the checklist in Chapter 1.
5. While there are many good reasons to sell your practice to a hospital, they do not include a big buyout and long-term salary guarantee.
6. Hospitals aren't purchasing practices for altogether altruistic reasons. They need physicians to maintain and grow market share, support service lines, and show third-party payors they have an extensive network of providers to serve the payors' patient base.
7. Hospitals need critical mass to "play" in the expected future bundled payment models, ACOs, PCMHs, and other initiatives.
8. Take a close look at the business viability of the hospital you are considering joining.
9. Make sure the hospital you choose is committed to making the necessary investment in physician practice management infrastructure and expertise.
10. Ask a lot of questions and be leery if you don't get straight answers. "We'll figure that out later" as the answer to most of your questions should be a red flag as to how well the hospital has thought through its strategy.
11. Consider how you would feel about answering to hospital administration.
12. Ask yourself what the hospital has to offer that will improve the quality of your professional and/or personal life. Then consider if what it is offering is enough for you to give up your autonomy. An attractive buyout price, a solid compensation and benefits package, fewer administrative hassles, and more time for direct patient care might align quite well with your long-term career values and goals.
13. It is not the hospital with the best offer that is likely to sustain you should you decide to sell—rather, it is the hospital with the commitment to practice management infrastructure, a solid business plan, and the successful execution of that plan.
14. Selling your practice should be pursued only after carefully considering an exit strategy if it doesn't work out.

Checklist: Initial Questions for the Hospital and Employed Physicians

❏ A hospital should take a healthy, proactive approach to practice acquisition. Ask about its reasons for buying practices. The answers you are looking for include the following:
  - Long-term strategy to grow or maintain market share;
  - Response to competitive threats;
  - Ability to better serve patients;
  - Strategic preparation for new payment models and integrated delivery;
  - Increased leverage in negotiation with third-party payors; and
  - Desire to help its medical staff members survive and thrive.

❏ Answers that should send up red flags might include the following:
  - Competitors are buying practices; and
  - Ability to cut your overhead.

❏ Ask a lot of questions about the hospital's practice management commitment and be cautious if you don't get specific answers:
  - How many physicians does the hospital currently employ?
  - How many practices does it plan to acquire?
  - How many physicians have left employment? Why?
  - What practice management expertise does the hospital currently have?
  - What practice management positions does the hospital anticipate adding in the future and/or what kind of background is it looking for to fill those positions?
  - How does it do, or plan to do, billing?
  - Does the hospital use provider-based billing charging patients a separate facility fee for an office visit?
  - Will billing be a centralized function, or will each practice keep its existing billing system?
  - Does it currently use or have plans for an EHR system?
  - Who will actually negotiate managed care contracts?
  - What is the hospital's business plan for practice acquisition and management?
  - How does my practice fit into that plan?
  - Will I have a say in the hiring and termination of staff?
  - How will staff work rules be enforced?
  - Will I have input into staff evaluations, raises, and bonuses?
  - Can my office be moved or consolidated with another office without my approval?

❑ Talk to physicians who have already gone through the acquisition process and ask these questions:
- How was it handled?
- Are they happy?
- Are they aware of unhappy physicians leaving?
- Has the hospital been willing to work with them to resolve problems and issues?

CHAPTER 5

Valuation—What Is Your Practice Worth?

Until you value yourself, you won't value your time. Until you value your time, you will not do anything with it.

M. SCOTT PECK

I f you decide to further explore the sale of your practice and see what your chosen hospital has to offer, the hospital will engage an independent firm—chosen and paid for by the hospital—to assess your practice and arrive at a fair market value. You will be asked to share extensive financial and operating data. Providing complete and accurate data is important. Incomplete documentation tends to reduce the value of a practice because absent documentation, the valuation firm is likely to make the most conservative assumptions. This is where the efforts you took in preparing your practice as discussed in Chapter 3 will start to pay off.

VALUATION COMPONENTS

The value of any business, including physician practices, generally consists of two types of assets: tangible and intangible.

Tangible assets in a physician practice consist of furniture and equipment, inventory and supplies, and accounts receivable (A/R). Many practices also own the practice's facility, often through a separate real estate entity that leases the facility to the practice.

Intangible assets include things like an established patient base, reputation of the physician(s), an established referral base, a trained workforce, patient medical records, and the name and phone number of the practice. Intangible assets are often referred to as "goodwill."

A valuation worksheet at the end of this chapter will assist you in estimating the value of your practice for comparison to the hospital's valuation.

VALUATION OF TANGIBLE ASSETS

Furniture and Equipment

Furniture and equipment will be valued at less than your original cost but probably more than their current net book value for tax purposes, which is simply the original cost less the total depreciation you have been allowed to deduct on your tax return since you purchased the asset.

Tax law generally allows depreciating assets over a fairly short period of time—generally a much shorter time than the actual period the asset will be used in the practice—therefore, net book value is probably going to understate the actual value of your furniture and equipment.

The appraisers will ask for or take a physical inventory that lists all the furniture and equipment in your practice, including description, make and model, date acquired, and original cost of the major items. Sometimes this information can be obtained from a depreciation schedule, which is a work paper your CPA firm maintains for use in preparing your tax return. Depreciation schedules are often incomplete and out of date, so make sure you review yours and update it as needed. If the appraiser asks you to complete a physical inventory, take the time to provide complete and accurate information.

The value of furniture and equipment is generally determined through secondary market prices or as a percent of what is called standard replacement cost.

The value of items that are of a more specialized nature, such as exam tables, and expensive medical equipment, such as x-ray and ultrasound machines or lab and other diagnostic or treatment equipment, is often determined based on the secondary or used equipment market. The Internet provides easy access to dozens of used-equipment vendors as well as other marketplaces such as eBay. These items are generally valued at the prices for which functionally similar equipment is for sale or recently sold in the secondary market.

Items of a more generic nature that are not readily available in the secondary market are often valued at a percent of standard replacement cost. Standard replacement cost is the appraiser's estimate of the replacement cost of furnishing a physician office with equipment of like utility. The value is generally a percent of the standard replacement cost based on the age and condition of your furniture and equipment.

A rule of thumb that can be used to estimate the value of a practice's furniture and equipment is to take net book value and add back 50% of the accumulated depreciation shown on your balance sheet. Your CPA can help you with this calculation if necessary, or you can try it yourself using the worksheet at the end of this chapter. While this method will not be totally accurate, it will give you a rough idea of the value to expect.

Make sure you exclude from your estimate, assets that tend to be more personal in nature. The hospital likely won't be interested in purchasing any antique furniture, original artwork, or practice-owned vehicles.

Finally, be sure to disclose equipment that is in need of repairs, even though it may be tempting to avoid doing so. You don't want to get your relationship with your new hospital partners off to a bad start over a small issue with equipment. The belief you were deliberately misleading the hospital in the sales process could easily translate into the belief that you will mislead the hospital on other issues as well.

Accounts Receivable (A/R)

Accounts receivable represents work you've already done and, while a tangible asset of your practice, is usually not part of the transaction. If a hospital does purchase A/R, which is rare, it will do so at a discounted rate and then attempt to collect (and keep) what it gets post-sale. In most instances, it's better for both parties if the physician keeps the outstanding A/R. Hospitals will usually allow your billing staff, who become their employees after the sale, to spend some time each week for a few months collecting your A/R.

A rule of thumb for estimating the value of A/R is to take the total balance of A/R outstanding less than 60 days and multiply it by your practice's historical gross collection rate. In most practices, the value should be equal to between one and two months' worth of collections. Here again, this method will not be totally accurate, but it will give you a rough idea of the value to expect.

The collection of these accounts receivable after the sale results in a kind of "bonus" to physicians selling their practice. You will be paid a salary by the hospital and also realize additional income through the collection of the A/R. Some savvy physicians and physician groups I have worked with who are skeptical about working for a hospital have decided to set aside the collections from their A/R as a sort of rainy-day fund to provide a ready source of working capital should they ever decide to go back into private practice. While there are tax implications of this strategy that should be discussed with your CPA, one of the biggest barriers to hospital-employed physicians restarting private practice is funding the working capital needed during the accounts receivable ramp-up period. Avoiding the temptation to spend these funds can be a sound strategy.

Inventory and Supplies

Inventory and supplies generally are not a significant component of the tangible value. If you have an extensive inventory of drugs and supplies, it will be to your benefit to provide copies of recent invoices to aid the hospital in assigning a fair value to these items. Don't attempt to enhance your value by trying to sell expired vaccines and drugs at full price: the hit on your reputation and future relationships are not worth the few extra dollars gained.

The rule of thumb here is to estimate the value by adding your average annual costs for office and medical supplies and drugs and multiplying by .17. This equates to about two months' worth of annual expense in inventory, which again, should provide a reasonable estimate.

Real Estate

Many practices own their own office building, generally as an entity separate from the practice entity. This asset, while not technically part of your practice's value, often represents the majority of your investment and is a key consideration in your decision to sell.

Many hospitals simply will not purchase physician-owned real estate. Instead, they will offer to lease the office space at a fair market value rental rate. If this is the hospital's approach, be sure the lease term is long enough to adequately provide you with a rental income stream to cover any mortgage payments and that there is clear agreement on things like taxes, insurance, repairs, and maintenance.

Some hospitals will purchase real estate, especially if it is located in a desirable location. Here, too, the hospital will engage an independent third-party appraiser (often a different appraiser than the one who valued the practice) and will be bound by the appraiser's valuation. If you don't feel the appraisal reflects the fair value of the facility or, as has often been the case in recent years, you feel the value is depressed as a result of the economy, leasing the facility to the hospital for a few years with a "put" option can provide the best of both worlds. A put option requires the hospital to purchase the office at some future date for its appraised value at that time.

Another option that many hospitals offer is to put you in touch with a third-party investor or real estate developer who might purchase your real estate.

VALUATION OF INTANGIBLE ASSETS

The value of tangible assets, with the exception of real estate, usually does not represent the bulk of what a physician thinks the practice is worth. Most physicians have the expectation of value in the intangible assets or what is commonly known as goodwill.

Physicians tend to think their practices are worth more than they actually are. The first argument is usually how much revenue the practice generates for the hospital by admitting patients and making referrals for diagnostic testing and therapeutic care. This is an easy one to set aside: It is illegal for a hospital to factor this in, and no reputable hospital would do so.

The second argument is that there has to be value in the practice's goodwill. After all, returning patients, the reputation of the doctors, trained providers and staff, an established referral base, medical records, and even the name and phone number of the practice are what make the practice a viable business, so those things have to have value.

While this goodwill does exist, the reality is that in the sale of a practice, it often has little or no value. This is because that value is almost always paid out to the physician owners in salary and bonus annually, and this will generally continue after the sale. The value of almost any business is in the future earnings stream that the business can be expected to generate for its owner. In this case, the owner will be the hospital. If the earnings stream the practice generates for the hospital is paid out to the physicians in salary and bonus, then, the theory goes, there is no earnings stream on which to base the value.

Another way to think of this is that you are, in effect, benefiting from the goodwill of the practice each year through the earnings it generates for you.

INCOME APPROACH

The income approach is usually developed on what is called the discounted cash flow (DCF) method. While the name may sound complex, the DCF method is really quite simple. The appraiser will develop a projection of the future financial performance of the practice, usually for a period of five years. This financial projection consists of three key components: revenue, practice overhead, and provider compensation.

Any projected future earnings (after physician compensation) are discounted to the present to arrive at the value—hence the term "discounted" cash flow. The discount simply reflects the time value of money (because a dollar in the future is worth less in today's dollars) and the risk inherent in attaining the future projected cash flow. The resulting number or DCF value represents what is often referred to as the business enterprise value or total value of the practice.

Under the income approach, the intangible value is often expressed simply as the excess of this business enterprise value over and above the value of the tangible assets of the practice. The valuation worksheet at the end of this chapter should help you understand the relationships and how they will impact the value of your practice.

This is where your revenue and overhead are normalized based on your practice's historical performance and current situation. The hospital won't pay you in upfront value for improvements it plans to make to augment the performance of the practice, such as better billing and collections, more favorable payor contracts, or overhead reductions. You will want to make sure that your incentive compensation (see Chapter 6) doesn't penalize you if the changes the hospital implements don't work out and result in decreased revenue, increased overhead, and decreased earnings.

The DCF method is the reason that demonstrating a healthy financial picture is important. Showing a healthy annual increase in revenue for the past year or two will support projecting a higher rate of revenue growth in the future. This may translate into a higher revenue projection that could result in a higher earnings stream and DCF value. Conversely, historical overhead that increases at stable or low rates will support lower expense projections.

Regardless of the projections, provider compensation makes or breaks a valuation using the DCF method. Historically, the earnings stream in almost all medical practices is paid out to the owners of the practice in the form of salary and bonuses. If the financial projections assume the physicians continue to be paid 100% of the funds available after overhead, there will be no value for the practice beyond the value of the furniture, fixtures, and equipment. Stated another way: If your post-sale compensation is projected to be equal to or greater than what you have historically earned, your practice is likely to have no value using the DCF method.

The physician compensation used in the valuation model ultimately should be based on your projected compensation as a hospital employee.

While the prospect that your practice may have no goodwill value using the income approach may be surprising and disappointing, if you step back and think about it, it makes sense. Why would anyone purchase a practice without a reasonable expectation of generating a profit from its operation? As noted above, the hospital cannot consider the value of any referrals because that would squarely be at odds with federal law.

So if you want to maintain your current income and get a big price for your practice, prepare to be disappointed. *Continuing 100% of your historical earnings post-acquisition may leave no future earnings for the value to be based on, in which case there may be no value beyond the value of your individual assets.*

If the compensation you ultimately negotiate (Chapter 6) is higher than the compensation used in the DCF model to value your practice, the value of your practice may actually go down. As noted above, the DCF model needs to accurately reflect the compensation that will be paid to the physician post-sale, including an estimate of incentive compensation. So the valuation model is often recalculated based on the agreed-upon salary and incentive structure, and the value will go up or down as a result. *This is the inverse relationship between practice value and post-sale compensation—higher salary equals lower value, and lower salary equals higher value.*

It may be possible to increase the value of your practice by agreeing to put a portion of your compensation at risk, that is, by agreeing to a lower salary. For example, you may agree to a salary of $25,000 less per year. The result will be an increase in the earnings stream of $25,000 per year in the DCF projection model, which may lead to a higher practice value.

This may sound like a good deal, but generally it is not. Your base salary could end up locked in at the lower level for several years, and subject to productivity standards (see Chapter 6). As noted above, any incentive compensation has to be estimated and included in the valuation model as well. There are tax implications that may need to be considered, too. So while some hospitals may consider this model, at the end of the day, most hospitals will shy away from such a structure because they don't want to be paying huge upfront values.

Entire books have been written on valuing physician practices. Practice brokers and dozens of firms are on the Internet offering to tell you, for a price or commission, what your practice is worth and to help you sell it. If you are going to sell to a hospital, don't bother with these services. It doesn't matter what these firms tell you. The hospital is going to be bound by the value determined by its independent appraiser and no more.

Another poor source of information on the value of your practice is the Internet. We recently were asked to value a practice owned by two nurse practitioners. They told the hospital that, "according to their Internet research," their practice was worth $1 million. While it turned out to be a robust practice with good financial performance, it still had no value using the income approach and therefore no goodwill value.

Historically many hospitals, both for-profit and not-for-profit, have taken an even more conservative approach: They simply have a policy against paying for intangible assets or goodwill—period. In many areas of the country, especially in the early stages of the current practice acquisition/sale trend, physicians were approaching hospitals—which indicated that in these areas it was a buyer's market. In a buyer's market, there is no compelling reason to pay for intangible assets or goodwill regardless of the practice's value. While this trend is still present in many markets, as further discussed below, in some markets this is changing.

Even in areas where there is competition among hospitals for practices, CEOs and hospital board members remember the lessons from the 1990s. Many simply are not willing to expose their hospital (or their job security) to repeating past mistakes.

To get a better value for your practice, properly prepare your practice for sale (Chapter 3) and focus on the things that matter: a demonstrated ability to earn well above the regional average for your specialty, a solid history of revenue growth, and a willingness to put part of your historical compensation at risk based on the future performance of the practice.

ANCILLARY SERVICES

Practices that provide ancillary services often want to treat these services as a separate business during the valuation process. Their argument is that if the provision of CT scans through an imaging center is generating a profit, for example, that earnings stream has a separate and discrete value.

While ancillary services can generate a significant profit for a physician practice, many physicians tend to overstate the income they generate. Ancillary services provided through the physician practice are essentially operating as a department within the practice.

The nature of practice accounting systems is that the "profit" generated doesn't fully reflect the cost of operating the ancillary service. Scheduling and billing are two common examples of services that are generally provided by the practice but whose costs are not separately allocated and reflected in internal financial reports. So the profit from the CT imaging would be significantly less if it were truly a standalone business.

An even more significant issue in valuing in-office ancillary services is one that physicians often forget: *The ancillary profits, however they are calculated, are already reflected in physician incomes from the practice and therefore are already reflected in the practice's valuation.*

Physicians seeking to maintain their current income post-sale and get a separate buyout for their CT business are double-dipping. Their incomes already include profits from the CT imaging. Therefore, that earnings stream has no discrete value to the hospital purchaser, because the physician is already taking the profits as part of his or her compensation.

To make matters even worse, these services are generally characterized by high fixed costs, so ongoing reimbursement cuts for these services have a disproportionate impact on the earnings stream they generate. The appraiser will project future earnings from these services based on projected future (practice, not hospital) reimbursement rates. I have seen many examples where the projected profitability of a service virtually disappears in the wake of reimbursement cuts.

VALUATION TRENDS

Even the highly regulated healthcare marketplace is subject to market pressures driven by the law of supply and demand. As noted above, the early stages of the current trend of hospitals acquiring physician practices was driven primarily by physicians. In many markets, this led to a buyer's market and allowed hospitals to hide behind policies of "no goodwill."

As happened in the 1990s, when competition among hospitals heated up, prices for physician practices started to rise. While hospitals cannot pay more than fair market value determined by an independent third-party appraiser, in some areas market competition has led to a relaxation of these "no goodwill" policies and given rise to valuation methodologies that seem to be at odds with one another.

In general terms, two opposing valuation theories are being used. One maintains what was stated above: if a business isn't projected to generate a positive future earnings stream then, by definition, it has no intangible asset value. Why, the theory goes, would a purchaser pay for value in excess of the tangible assets for a business that loses money?

The second theory maintains that the nature of a physician practice is that it provides a community benefit beyond what can be indicated by its future earnings. This value may be manifest in capacity, meaning a healthcare system is capable of fulfilling its mission by providing a full range of services and remaining sustainable under evolving future payment models. This is one of the major underpinnings of health reform. This second theory asks: How can an established practice, regardless of its income statement performance, not have any intangible value for its existence as an established center of healthcare for the community?

Without getting into complex valuation theory, this argument is usually based on the principle of substitution, which compares the cost of replicating the practice being purchased to a *de novo* startup of a practice. The cost of building an established patient base, trained workforce, and ongoing revenue stream is, at one level, the essence of intangible value.

As stated above, returning patients, the reputation of the doctors, trained providers and staff, an established referral base, medical records, and even the name and phone number of the practice are what make the practice a viable business, so those things have to have value.

We currently are seeing few hospitals pay for goodwill per se, but some are willing to pay for medical records and a trained workforce in place. Some hospitals that are paying for these assets are requiring a repurchase of them in the event the sale is unwound in the future and the physicians go back into private practice. The last thing a hospital wants is an asset on its books that it has to write down to a zero value if and when your employment arrangement ceases.

The disagreement between these two theories boils down to whether these things have value in the absence of a future earnings stream.

There are two important lessons here:

1. Valuation is part art and part science, and there are legitimate disagreements on these issues between highly trained and experienced experts on both sides.
2. Hospital policies on payment for intangible assets vary widely, and some hospitals are changing those policies out of competitive necessity in markets where competition for physician practices is heating up and the market is shifting from a buyer's market to more of a seller's market.

Where you come out and how this impacts the sale of your practice is unpredictable, and many nuances must be considered. For example, I recently was involved in a situation where a solo family practitioner was making a strong case, through his practice consultant, that his staff had significant value as a "trained workforce in place." A simple review of his practice's employee salary levels and turnover refuted this assertion because the quality of his staff members was reflected in their low salaries, lack of experience, and high turnover.

Contrast this situation to a larger group down the street that employed a practice administrator with 15 years of experience, an MBA, and certification from the American College of Medical Practice Executives. The billing manager was a certified coder, and the midlevel providers had extensive experience in their specialty. Which practice would be more likely to demonstrate a value for its trained workforce?

Making specious claims about intangible value, or relying on some half-baked article off the Internet and adhering to a position unsupported by the facts can lead to a loss of respect by hospital administration. One hospital I was working with pointed out that the value a physicians' group wanted assigned to its workforce went against the hospital's acquisition experience. The hospital had to replace 15% to 20% of the personnel in its previous acquisition because of the staff's lack of training and general inability to function as part of a larger organization.

HOSPITAL PERSPECTIVE

In spite of what you might assume, the hospital likely isn't trying to lowball you on the value of your practice or in your post-sale compensation. Many hospitals are willing to pay the full value of your practice as determined by the outside independent valuation firm. They are not willing to overpay for your practice because that would be illegal. While many hospitals are not willing to pay for goodwill or intangible value, regardless of the valuation, as a matter of policy, this is changing in some areas. Yet the controversy over intangible value when there is a lack of projected future earnings is unlikely to be definitively resolved in the immediate future.

The hospital wants you to be financially successful post-sale. It wants you to be happy and doesn't care if your income increases substantially as long as the hospital doesn't have significant losses on your practice. Here, too, an almost universal unwillingness to lose money on employing physicians that was prevalent a few years ago (which was largely a result of hospital experiences in the 1990s) has given way to a levels of losses that have gone well beyond what was expected and may be unsustainable.

TAKEAWAY POINTS FOR CHAPTER 5

1. The hospital will engage an independent firm, chosen and paid for by the hospital, to assess your practice and to arrive at a fair market value.
2. Providing complete and accurate data is important. Absent documentation, the valuation firm is likely to make the most conservative assumptions.
3. Physicians tend to think their practices are worth more than they actually are.
4. The value of any business generally consists of two types of assets: tangible and intangible.
5. Tangible assets consist of furniture and equipment, inventory and supplies, and A/R.
6. Intangible assets include things like an established patient base, reputation of the physician(s), trained providers and staff, an established referral base, patient

medical records, and the name and phone number of the practice. Intangible assets are often referred to as goodwill.

7. The valuation of tangible assets and how they are handled in a hospital sale are fairly standard. Furniture and equipment will be valued less than your original cost but probably more than their current net book value.

8. Usually the physician will keep the outstanding A/R, and the hospital will allow your billing staff to collect it post-sale.

9. Many hospitals will not purchase physician-owned real estate. Instead the hospital will enter into a space lease at fair market value rental rates. Be sure the lease terms are adequate and there is clear agreement on things like taxes, insurance, repairs, and maintenance.

10. Most physicians have the expectation of value in the intangible assets or what is commonly known as goodwill. There is currently disagreement between the two competing valuation methodologies as to whether intangible value exists in the absence of a future earnings stream. The intangible assets that are most often valued and acquired are medical records and a trained workforce in place.

11. Showing a healthy annual increase in revenue could result in a higher value.

12. If you want to maintain your current income and get a big price for your practice, prepare to be disappointed.

13. Ancillary profits are already reflected in physician incomes and, therefore, are already reflected in the practice's valuation.

14. Many hospitals are willing to pay the full value for your practice and don't care how much you earn. What they seek to do is to keep losses from employing physicians at controllable levels and the current market is experiencing losses that may be unsustainable.

15. Many hospitals simply are not willing to pay for intangible assets or goodwill value, regardless of the valuation, as a matter of policy, but market conditions are resulting in changes in this policy in some parts of the country.

PRACTICE VALUATION WORKSHEETS

These worksheets provide a simple tool for estimating the value of your practice. These are estimates only and likely will vary from the hospital's valuation. They should be used to highlight differences between the actual value of your practice and your estimate and as an aid in raising questions for discussion with the hospital.

Tangible Assets

Furniture, Fixtures and Equipment (FF&E)	Practice Estimate	Hospital Value
Cost		
– Accumulated depreciation		
= Net book value		
+ 50% of accumulated depreciation		
= Estimated Value of FF&E		

Accounts Receivable	Practice Estimate	Hospital Value
Accounts receivable outstanding less than 60 days		
– Practice's gross collection percentage (See Chapter 3 for definition)		
= Estimated Value of Accounts Receivable		

Inventory and Supplies	Practice Estimate	Hospital Value
Office supplies expense last year		
+ Medical supplies expense last year		
+ Vaccine and drug expense last year		
= Total drug and supply expense		
× Total by .1667 = Estimated Value		

Business Enterprise or Total Practice Value	Practice Estimate	Hospital Value
Practice revenue last year		
– True practice overhead last year (see Chapter 3, Income/Overhead Percentage Worksheet)		
– Post-sale provider compensation × 1.15 (including employed and midlevel providers)		
= Practice earnings		
= Total Estimated Practice Value		

Practice Value Summary	Practice Estimate	Hospital Value
Total Estimated Practice Value		
– Estimated Value of FF&E		
– Estimated Value of Accounts Receivable		
× Estimated Value of Inventory and Supplies		
= Goodwill Value (if negative number, goodwill value is zero)		

Intangible Assets

Note: Some hospitals will pay for the intangible assets listed below. Many will not under any circumstances. Some hospitals will not pay for intangible assets unless the practice has a positive value as determined by the income approach.

Medical Records	Practice Estimate	Hospital Value
Number of Active Patient Charts (patients seen within the past 12 months)		
× $15.00 = Estimated Value		

Trained Workforce in Place	Practice Estimate	Hospital Value
Total Salary and Benefit Costs (exclude physician owners but include employed physicians and midlevel providers)		
× 20% = Estimated Value		

CHAPTER 6

Compensation

Post-sale compensation is by far the most important financial aspect of selling your practice but, as many unhappy employed physicians have found, while compensation may be a primary consideration when selling, it generally isn't enough to overcome day-to-day dissatisfaction. If you have chosen your potential hospital partner wisely, you should have every expectation that your practice income will stabilize or even increase—just don't expect the compensation to be an end in itself.

This is an area where you can't ask too many questions and where involvement of your CPA or practice advisor is highly recommended. Compensation plans can be quite complex and you need to understand where the numbers come from and how the calculations are made. Don't be afraid to ask for examples and language clarification. Insist on sample illustrations of compensation calculations.

THE RISING ROLE OF FAIR MARKET VALUE

The attitude of hospitals toward physician compensation changed dramatically in the months following the August 25, 2009, announcement that Covenant Medical Center and Wheaton Franciscan Healthcare-Iowa, Inc., in Waterloo, Iowa, entered into a $4.5 million settlement agreement with the Department of Justice. The settlement was the resolution of an allegation that Covenant submitted false claims for services, because the compensation paid to its employed physicians exceeded fair market value and was not commercially reasonable.

Up to this time, most healthcare attorneys had assumed that hospital employment of physicians was a relatively safe way, from a regulatory standpoint, to align hospitals and physicians because regulations provide a statutory exception and safe harbors for employees. These exceptions, however, do require that compensation be consistent with fair market value and be commercially reasonable even if no referrals are made.

This investigation and settlement was among the first to focus exclusively on fair market value and commercially reasonable compensation paid to employed physicians by hospitals and have had far-reaching effects in the industry. As a result, most hospitals are obtaining third-party fair market value and commercial reasonableness opinions on most employed physician compensation arrangements.

"Fair market value" is defined as the compensation that would be included in a service agreement as the result of bona fide bargaining between well-informed parties who are not otherwise in a position to generate business for the other party. All compensation must be considered in determining fair market value, including salary, bonus, and benefits.

Most third parties providing fair market value compensation opinions feel most comfortable with compensation tied to productivity measured by wRVUs and benchmarked against surveys such as the MGMA Physician Compensation and Production Survey (Chapter 3). They feel this is the safest way to avoid regulatory scrutiny; as a result, there has been a dramatic industry shift away from other productivity metrics to an almost universal use of wRVUs. In addition, most independent appraisers and hospital legal counselors are also requiring caps on compensation levels.

When selling your practice, this might be an area where the survey biases discussed in Chapter 3 work to your benefit. Know what the median compensation is for your specialty based on the survey data, and if it is higher than what you are currently earning, you can always push for the increase.

COMPENSATION PLANS

Hospital compensation plans generally include multiple components or "buckets." Typical components include the following, which are each discussed in more detail below:

- Base salary;
- Incentive compensation;
- Nonproductivity incentives; and
- Other income.

Base Salary

The employment agreement often will provide for a base salary; the base salary often will be based on your historical earnings or a projection of your earnings under the hospital's compensation model or some combination of the two.

As discussed in Chapter 3, make sure the historical earnings actually reflect the earning potential of the practice and that your historical income has been adjusted for physician discretionary expenses.

Think of base salary as the "bridge" between your historical income and your future income under the hospital's compensation plan—your assurance that if you maintain your work effort, your compensation will not decrease regardless of the terms of the hospital's compensation plan.

Base salary is sometimes negotiable, but remember, a higher base salary may result in a downward adjustment in the value of your practice in certain situations because of the inverse relationship between practice value and compensation, which was discussed in Chapter 5.

Usually the base salary is guaranteed for a period of time, usually no longer than one or two years. This period can sometimes be negotiated as well, but most employment contracts still require that some level of productivity be maintained to earn the base salary.

Productivity Standards

During the early stages of the current cycle of hospital employment of physicians (See Chapter 1), base salaries were almost universally subject to productivity standards based on wRVUs. This was a reflection of both the fair market value concerns discussed above and the productivity declines that tended to result in the absence of such standards. However, we have begun seeing transactions in which productivity standards are absent, and this trend seems to be expanding.

As alternative payment models emerge, many feel that productivity standards such as wRVUs, which incentivize volume, will need to give way to other measures. This may be true in the future, but establishing those metrics now is virtually impossible until the underlying metrics are defined by the payors and can be measured.

Regardless of the productivity standard, it is important to understand how the historical data were determined and that this is comparable to how it will be calculated in the future.

The typical contract will offer you a base salary that is contingent on maintaining a specified productivity standard similar to what you have produced historically.

For example, if you had 8,000 wRVUs last year, the standard may be that you agree to maintain wRVUs of no less than 90%—or 7,200 wRVUs—to earn your base salary. If your wRVUs fall below that number, there may be a prorated reduction in your base salary. So if your base salary is, for example, $240,000 and your wRVUs drop by 10%, your base salary may drop by 10% to $216,000. Often there is a "fudge factor" that allows for some minor level of reduced productivity before compensation is reduced.

If you completed the steps in preparing your practice for sale outlined in Chapter 3, you should already have an accurate determination of your historical wRVUs.

This should make it fairly easy to assess how your compensation will fare under the compensation plan being proposed by the hospital.

As noted in Chapter 3, many physician billing systems do not provide wRVU data, and, when they do, they are often based on outdated wRVU values. wRVU values can and do change, so you want to be sure the wRVU data used by the hospital or its consultants accurately reflect your productivity. Since wRVU values will likely change in the future, make sure you understand how your productivity standard will be adjusted to reflect these future changes.

While wRVUs have become the productivity standard of choice in most situations, other productivity standards still in use in some areas and situations include those discussed below.

Patient encounters

This is the most basic productivity standard. The main pitfalls with patient-encounter thresholds are defining an encounter and ensuring the accuracy of the historical patient-encounter data from which the standard is derived.

Physician billing systems often do not provide ready access to encounter data, and such data often have to be manually extracted by CPT code. There are also varying definitions of what exactly constitutes a patient encounter.

For example, do the data include encounters of a midlevel provider that were billed incident-to under the physician's name? How is time spent on midlevel provider supervision accounted for? What about nursing-only visits or rechecks that are billed under the physician's name? Practices handle these issues in varying ways. Finding that one definition was used in developing the standard and that another one is used by the hospital in evaluating the standard post-sale will result in problems down the road. It will always be beneficial to deal with these detail-type issues up front to avoid problems later.

Sometimes, especially in cases where midlevel provider visits are billed incident-to under a physician's name, accurate encounter data simply are not available. In this case, it may be necessary to manually determine encounters from an appointment schedule or log or agree to use a different standard.

Gross charges

Gross charges are a fair reflection of physician work effort from year to year only so long as the fee schedule on which they are based is consistent. Many practices are lax in updating their fee schedules. Hospitals, especially those experienced in practice management, will typically update fee schedules regularly based on national or regional norms, which can result in apples-to-oranges comparisons.

Cash collections

Some hospitals, especially those with little or no experience in the employment of physicians, will seek to minimize downside risk by attempting to measure productivity based on collections. Depending on how billing and collections functions are handled post-sale, this introduces a variable into the equation that you may not be able to control: the hospital's ability to bill and collect.

Using cash collections as a productivity standard can have an upside for physicians as well, because if the hospital does a better job of billing and collections or has better payor contracts, the physician will realize the benefit without any additional effort.

Hospitals with successful experience in practice management tend to have billing and collections down to a science. They often have invested heavily in technology, systems, and experienced personnel, and have top-tier billing offices. The trick is figuring out if your chosen hospital knows what it is doing before you agree to a cash collections productivity standard.

Regardless of the productivity standard used, you will want to be sure the definition of the standard is included in the contract language and that the definition is consistent with how your historical data were used to calculate the standard. In other words, make sure the productivity standard is calculated the same way on the front- and the back-end.

Incentive Compensation

Incentive compensation is one of the most important components of your post-sale employment. In light of the Waterloo settlement, incentive compensation has also evolved toward almost universal reliance on wRVUs.

Many variations come into play, but the basic mechanism is that incentive compensation is earned by producing wRVUs in excess of a predetermined threshold, and those excess wRVUs are multiplied by a dollar amount, usually referred to as a conversion factor, to determine the incentive compensation amount.

For instance, in the example above, where the productivity standard to earn the base salary of $240,000 was 8,000 wRVUs, or $30 per wRVU, the compensation plan might provide for a conversion factor of $35 on wRVUs in excess of 8,000.

Sometimes multiple tiers like the one in the above example are used. Some plans tie the conversion factor to productivity percentiles based on the MGMA survey, and that factor increases incrementally each time the next higher threshold is reached. A simple example of a multi-tiered incentive compensation plan is provided at the end of this chapter.

There are various permutations depending on the specific situation and what the hospital is trying to accomplish through its compensation plan. Two of the most common motivating factors that underlie a vast majority of wRVU-based incentive compensation plans offered by hospitals are:

1. They want to incentivize incremental wRVUs because the fixed-cost nature of a medical practice means that the revenue generated by the incremental wRVUs comes without a material increase in overhead costs. So the additional incentive compensation resulting from higher levels of production still increases the hospital's operating margin or reduces the hospital's operating losses.
2. They feel that incentive compensation based on additional productivity (i.e., work) is the safest way to avoid regulatory scrutiny and meet fair market value tests.

The weaknesses of an incentive compensation plan based solely on wRVUs include the following:

1. There is no incentive for the physician to control costs.
2. The wRVUs become a "currency" that has value to the physicians regardless of whether they produce any revenue for the hospital. One example would be wRVUs generated on indigent patients. While the hospital may want to provide indigent care as part of its mission, paying physicians to generate wRVUs that produce no corresponding revenue is not a business model that will be sustainable in the long run.

Some compensation plans use incentives other than wRVUS as described below, although these are less common in the aftermath of the Waterloo settlement.

Virtual Private Practice and Profit-based Incentives. The virtual private practice (VPP) model attempts to replicate the economics of private practice in an employed physician environment. In its basic form under the VPP model, the physicians are compensated based solely on the earnings of the practice.

Profit-based incentives are similar to the VPP model except the profit only affects incentive (or bonus) compensation. This was once a common type of incentive plan because it, by its very nature, limits hospital losses on physician practices. Profit-based incentives don't prevent hospitals from losing money but, without profits, the hospital isn't obligated to pay incentive compensation, which limits its downside.

Profit-based incentives are generally not available for use by not-for-profit hospitals unless a for-profit subsidiary can be established. Even in that case, hospital legal counsel often will insist compensation be subject to a cap.

Hospitals make VPP and profit-based incentive plans attractive because they protect the hospital's downside. Hospitals typically offer a high percentage of profits to the physicians: 50% is common for an incentive plan, but I've seen the incentive percentages go as high as 90%. With the VPP model, the physicians generally receive 100% of the earnings of the practice.

The key issue with both of these models is in the definition of "profit." Is it revenue based on cash collections? If so, the ability of the hospital to bill and collect has to be considered, as discussed above. Often, as noted in Chapter 9, revenue is recorded on an accrual basis, which relies on estimates of future collections that may be of questionable accuracy—especially in the early stages of employment where sufficient historical data is not available to provide for accurate estimates.

Does overhead include an allocation for the hospital's management infrastructure and such things as accounting, payroll processing, billing, IT and administration? While allocation of direct costs is reasonable, some hospitals, especially those inexperienced in practice management, will allocate administrative overhead and other costs well in excess of the fair value of the services provided.

Some hospitals will attempt to allocate the depreciation and amortization of the purchase price paid for the practice. While allocation of depreciation expense on tangible assets is reasonable, allocating the amortization of goodwill (in instances where it exists) ensures ongoing operating losses.

VPP and profit-based incentives can be lucrative to physicians, and they are effective in aligning incentives between the physicians and the hospital but, are also full of potential pitfalls that must be considered.

Enterprise Incentives. Enterprise incentives are more typically used by not-for-profit hospitals that cannot establish a for-profit subsidiary and seek a way to provide an effective incentive plan within the confines of their not-for-profit structure.

These plans tend to be complex, but they generally seek to establish an incentive based on the hospital's employed physicians, as a group, attaining certain financial and operational goals. While these plans can be very lucrative, they effectively put incentive compensation out of the direct control of individual physicians and rely instead on broader goals and group-wide objectives.

This type of incentive has the tendency to be frustrating to high-performing physicians because they can be penalized for the inability of others to contribute to the team effort.

Other Variations. There are hybrid incentive compensation plans combining, on some basis, two or more of the above components. The possibilities are limited only by the imagination and the limits of fair market value.

Whatever the compensation plan, ask a lot of questions and ask to see sample—or even actual—calculations in cases where the incentive has been in use with other practices. Ask how the incentive has been realized in the past. Talk to other physicians who have operated under the plan to gauge their satisfaction.

Nonproductivity Incentives

The third component of compensation is often nonproductivity or "quality" incentives, which have, in the light of health reform, become an increasingly common component of compensation plans.

Many physicians like to think of these incentives as a way to increase their compensation without additional work effort, but in reality this is usually not the case.

For fair market value testing purposes, nonproductivity incentive compensation is generally assumed to be earned and must be included in total compensation. Median quality is generally assumed as part of base salary and incentive compensation. So quality and other nonproductivity incentives usually represent additional "stretch goals" and generally require additional effort on the part of the physicians.

These incentives can be based on achievement of quality metrics by individual physicians, specialty, group, or some combination of these. Metrics often vary by specialty, and some tend to be private practice oriented while others can be more hospital oriented.

How the metrics are defined, monitored, measured, and applied requires careful consideration. For example, if all nonproductivity incentives are based on achievement by all physicians in your specialty, you could find your compensation adversely affected in spite of your efforts to meet the standards. In addition, some nonproductivity incentives are "pass/fail," and others provide for partial payment in cases where the metrics are partially achieved.

Typically these incentives are 5% to 10% of total compensation. Most experts feel that quality incentives are an important part of modern compensation plan design and that this percentage will increase in the future as the delivery of healthcare evolves and the technology available to monitor the metrics becomes more prevalent.

Other Income

Other income typically encompasses a broad spectrum of additional amounts paid to physicians. As with other forms of compensation, other income typically has to be included in the fair market value testing. Examples include hospital stipends for department chairs, medical directorships, call pay, and moonlighting in the emergency department.

To the extent these payments existed prior to you becoming an employee of the hospital, be sure you understand how and whether they will continue in the future.

TAKEAWAY POINTS FOR CHAPTER 6

1. Post-sale compensation is by far the most important financial aspect of selling your practice.

2. The attitude of hospitals toward physician compensation changed dramatically following the Department of Justice allegation that a hospital in Waterloo, Iowa, paid compensation to its employed physicians in excess of fair market value.

3. The Waterloo settlement has moved many hospitals to require third-party fair market value opinions on most employed physician compensation arrangements and has also resulted in a movement toward compensation based on wRVUs.

4. The employment agreement typically provides for a base salary, likely based on your historical earnings. Usually the base salary is guaranteed for a period of time, usually no longer than one or two years, but still will include productivity standards.

5. Typical hospital compensation plans include components for base salary, incentive compensation, quality incentives, and other income.

6. Think of base salary as a bridge between your historical income and your future income under the hospital's compensation plan.

7. Base salaries are almost universally subject to productivity standards based on sRVUs except in the VPP model.

8. Incentive compensation is one of the most important components of your post-sale employment.

9. The weaknesses of a productivity-based incentive from the hospital's perspective are that it provides no incentive for the physicians to control costs and that producing wRVUs can enhance physician income without generating any corresponding revenue for the hospital.

10. Nonproductivity incentives have become an increasingly common component of compensation plans.

11. For fair market value testing purposes, nonproductivity incentive compensation is generally assumed to be earned and must be included in total compensation.

12. Median quality is generally assumed as part of base salary and incentive compensation. So such incentives usually represent additional stretch goals and generally require additional effort on the part of the physicians.

13. How the metrics are defined, monitored, measured, and applied requires careful consideration.

14. Typically nonproductivity incentives are 5% to 10% of total compensation but most experts feel that this percentage will increase in the future as the delivery of healthcare evolves and the technology available to monitor the metrics becomes more prevalent.

Multi-Tiered wRVU Compensation Plan Illustration

In this illustration, there are four productivity tiers based on the MGMA Production and Compensation Survey (see chart on the next page). A physician's compensation is his or her wRVUs multiplied by the conversion factor applicable to his or her production level.

Doctor 2 produced 4,810 wRVUs, which is just below the 50th percentile (median), so his compensation is based on a conversion factor of $37.50.

Doctor 3 produced 4,850 wRVUs, which is just above the 50th percentile (median), so her compensation is based on the higher conversion factor of $40.

So although these two physicians produced almost identical wRVUs, the compensation plan was designed to incentivize attaining higher levels of productivity, which resulted in disproportionately higher compensation for Doctor 3 over Doctor 2. This characteristic is common in plan design. Conversion factors and wRVU tiers generally vary by specialty.

Example of Multi-tiered Incentive Compensation Plan

Compensation Plan Parameters				
MGMA Percentile At Least	MGMA Percentile Not > Than	MGMA WRVUs At Least	MGMA WRVUs Not > Than	Conversion Factor
-0-	40th	—	4,497	$35.00
40th	50th	4,497	4,845	$37.50
50th	60th	4,845	5,194	$40.00
60th	70th	5,194	5,610	$45.50
70th		5,610		$45.00
Example Calculations				
	Actual WRVUs	Conversion Factor	Compensation	
Doctor 1	4,225	$35.00	$147,875	
Doctor 2	4,810	$37.50	$180,375	
Doctor 3	4,850	$40.00	$194,000	
Doctor 4	5,725	$45.00	$257,625	

CHAPTER 7

Deal Structure

Hospital acquisition of a physician practice generally consists of two components: an asset purchase agreement and an employment agreement. In some situations, there may be other agreements. For example, if real estate is being purchased, this would be subject to a separate real estate purchase agreement.

ASSET PURCHASE AGREEMENT

The asset purchase agreement is simply an agreement wherein you agree to sell and the hospital agrees to purchase specified practice assets for a specified price with specified payment terms. The assets included will vary but generally include all of the tangible furniture, fixtures, and equipment along with your inventory and supplies.

Asset purchase agreements also generally include intangible assets such as the practice's name, phone number, and patient records, even if a separate value is not assigned to these items. Many physicians question why they should agree to sell these items for little or no value. The answer is that these intangible assets are part of the practice, and most hospitals will insist on including them. You might think of this as the cost of getting the hospital to enter into the employment agreement discussed below.

Asset purchase agreements are usually pretty straightforward. You will attest you own the assets being sold and that they are free of liens or encumbrances. There generally will be a list of the assets. Review this list carefully and make sure any personal items, which often are present in physician offices, are excluded from the sale.

Any outstanding debt your practice has, including loans to purchase equipment or any loans secured by your practice's assets, generally will not be assumed by the hospital. You likely will need to make arrangements to pay these loans off and get any security interests released prior to closing.

Equipment and space leases probably will be assumed by the hospital. Generally, you will need to secure the permission of the equipment leasing company and your landlord prior to closing as well. While seeking such approvals is often considered a formality, it is possible for these details to delay closing, so it is best to identify these issues for the hospital in advance so its legal counsel can work on getting the necessary paperwork completed.

Asset purchase agreements often also will include a restrictive covenant or non-compete provision, which is discussed in detail below.

While you never want to plan for failure, consider whether you want a provision that states how you will purchase the assets back in the future. Sometimes the security of knowing how the assets will be revalued at some future date is comforting. Other times, you may be better off just leaving this to chance—after all, if the deal fails, the hospital may not want your old equipment, and you might get a better deal if the price or valuation method isn't stated.

As noted above, in situations where hospitals agree to acquire intangible assets such as medical records and trained workforce in place, some require the repurchase of these assets in the event of termination should you go back into private practice or otherwise want to obtain the medical records and hire back the staff. This is somewhat rare, but it is something you should be aware of in case the issue arises during the negotiations.

EMPLOYMENT AGREEMENT

The employment agreement is your agreement to become an employee of the hospital and sets out the employment terms, termination provisions, and the all-important compensation provisions including salary, incentive compensation, and benefits. The compensation plan of the hospital (Chapter 6) generally is included as an exhibit to the employment agreement and is often where physicians focus most of their effort.

The employment agreement is generally much more important than the asset purchase agreement. It specifies both parties' rights and obligations and otherwise governs your day-to-day work from now on. Make sure you fully understand its provisions. The employment agreement also should be given a detailed review by your attorney, who may raise additional questions and issues.

Beyond compensation, the following are some key provisions you should review and understand:

Termination with cause

Most employment agreements provide for termination with cause. "Cause" is usually defined to include such things as death, disability, and conviction of a felony. While some of these causes are easy to recognize, care needs to be taken when the determination is vague. For example, what is the definition of "disability"? How is it determined? Is there an appeals process?

Termination without cause

Sometimes both sides have done everything right, and it just doesn't work. Other times, unanticipated issues come up, and the parties need to compromise. Some hospitals, seeking to avoid these conflicts, offer termination without cause provisions. These provisions generally provide that either party, upon giving required notice (usually 90 to 180 days), can terminate the relationship for any reason.

How will you purchase your practice back? How will the price be determined, and under what terms will you be required to make payment? How will malpractice tail coverage be handled? Will the restrictive covenant be waived? Many hospitals are willing to waive the restrictive covenant in the case of termination if you return to private practice, but will want assurance that you will not sell or otherwise affiliate with one of their hospital competitors.

Finally, make sure the contract provides for an adequate notice time. While 180 days may seem like an eternity, once you've made the decision to go back on your own, you likely will need much of that time to get your provider numbers and payor contracts back in your name, reestablish billing and collections functions, transition staff back to your employment, and get the legal documentation completed.

Restrictive covenant (noncompete)

Most employment agreements (and some asset purchase agreements as noted above) will include some kind of restrictive covenant or noncompete provision. Restrictive covenants generally prohibit you from practicing medicine for a specified period of time within a specified distance of a geographic location such as the hospital or your office location.

While the idea of a restrictive covenant may seem offensive, absent a noncompete provision, your practice has less value to the hospital. Interestingly, we have seen situations where states have virtually outlawed noncompetes and other restrictive covenants with physicians. Physicians rejoiced, but that rejoicing was was short-lived when they discovered that the value hospitals were willing to pay for their practices decreased dramatically as a result. The ability of a purchaser to protect an asset is concomitant with the value, and removing that ability can have deleterious effect on that value.

Make sure the time, distance, and geographic location parameters of the noncompete are reasonable and practical. For example, a noncompete that restricts you from practicing within 20 miles of your practice location is less restrictive than one that prohibits you from practicing within 20 miles of any hospital-owned practice location.

These parameters are often negotiable and need to be considered in the context of your practice's service area, demographics, and competitive environment. These issues need to be considered carefully because you may be putting your future ability to practice in the area at risk if the relationship doesn't work out.

The enforceability and reasonableness of restrictive covenants are subject to state law and often complex legal precedents. As noted above, restrictive covenants are not enforceable in some states, and other states limit their enforceability to specific circumstances. Both of these situations can result in a reduction in what the hospital is willing to offer. Consult legal counsel with specific experience in this area.

Finally, relate the noncompete to the termination provisions. Generally you should try to negotiate that the noncompete should not apply if the contract is terminated for breach by the hospital or terminated by either party without cause (if the contract provides for such termination), or if the contract expires without renewal so long as you return to private practice. However, expect the hospital to take a fairly hard line on you becoming a "free agent" again and selling to a competing hospital.

Sign-on and retention bonuses

Some hospitals offer incentive payments to induce physicians to sell. These usually take the form of a sign-on or retention bonus and come in many variations. For example, sometimes the hospital will agree to pay a specified dollar amount upon the anniversary date of your employment for several years. Sometimes a certain percentage of your revenue, compensation, or bonus is set aside annually and paid in a lump sum after a specified period of time.

Retention bonuses are generally not prorated or paid in the event of early termination, but to the extent the hospital terminates the contract early, you may want to ask that payment be made.

Both sign-on and retention bonuses must be included in compensation for purposes of fair market value testing (Chapter 6). Consequently, they may result in offsetting decreases in base salary or incentive compensation and are appearing less frequently in employment agreements. They do, however, offer some distinct benefits to physicians in a sale and should not be overlooked in the negotiating process.

Severance

In the event of termination, you must understand any severance pay provisions. These are not common, and most contracts provide only for payment of base salary through the date of termination.

More important in the event of early termination is how trailing incentive compensation is handled. For example, if incentive compensation is calculated and paid quarterly, what happens if the contract is terminated two months into the quarter? Is the incentive calculation prorated, or are you simply out of luck?

Finally, consider how malpractice tail coverage will be handled in case of termination.

Governance, management, and day-to-day operational roles

Many physicians seek hospital employment so they can avoid being involved in day-to-day management, dealing with staff issues, and participating in group meetings and other governance activities. Some physicians, on the other hand, actually welcome involvement in these roles. As discussed in Chapter 1, involving physicians in governance has its problems, but either way, you want to be sure you understand what is required with respect to management and governance participation as part of the employment agreement and any potential impact these activities could have on your productivity and free time after hours.

Some hospitals set aside funds in their compensation plans to pay physicians who participate in governance, committee roles, and other management functions.

Unlike practice employment arrangements in the 1990s, when physicians were sold on the idea of "you just practice medicine," most hospital systems now believe it is necessary to engage physicians in governance and leadership roles.

Publicity

Many hospitals do not publicly announce or brand physicians as being part of the hospital. The approach to this issue varies greatly based on specific market competitive factors and even local custom. You may want to understand the hospital's strategy here, but don't expect too much control over how it chooses to promote or brand the practice.

TAKEAWAY POINTS FOR CHAPTER 7

1. Hospital acquisition of a physician practice generally consists of two components: an asset purchase agreement and an employment agreement.

2. Most employment agreements provide for termination with cause. Care needs to be taken in how "cause" is defined and who makes the determination.

3. Some hospitals, seeking to avoid these conflicts, offer termination without cause provisions. These provisions generally provide that either party, upon giving required notice (usually 90 to 180 days), can terminate the relationship for any reason.

4. Provisions for termination without cause often have the opposite effect. Rather than resulting in hasty termination, they provide the parties with a pathway to work together to resolve issues and strengthen the relationship.

5. Most employment agreements include some kind of restrictive covenant or noncompete provision. While this may seem offensive, absent a noncompete provision, your practice has no value to the hospital.

6. Time, distance, and geographic location parameters included in most restrictive covenants are often negotiable and should be considered in the context of your practice's service area, demographics, and competitive environment. These issues need to be considered carefully because you may be putting your ability to practice in the area in the future at risk if the relationship doesn't work out.

7. Some hospitals offer a sign-on or retention bonus. Both types of bonuses must be included in compensation for purposes of fair market value testing; consequently, this may result in an offsetting decrease in base salary or incentive compensation. While they are appearing less frequently in employment agreements, they have some distinct benefits and should not be overlooked in the negotiating process.

8. Many physicians seek hospital employment so they can avoid being involved in day-to-day management, dealing with staff issues, and participating in group meetings and other governance activities.

9. Unlike practice employment arrangements in the 1990s, when physicians were sold on the idea of "you just practice medicine," most hospital systems recognize the necessity of engaging physicians in governance and leadership roles. To better understand how these roles function, review Chapter 1.

CHAPTER 8

Negotiations

During a negotiation, it would be wise not to take anything personally. If you leave personalities out of it, you will be able to see opportunities more objectively. BRIAN KOSLOW

I f you've properly prepared your practice for sale as described in Chapter 3, you should have maximized your value and have a practice the hospital should be very interested in acquiring.

If you've done your homework as outlined in Chapter 4, you should have chosen a hospital that is financially stable and has a commitment to successful practice management.

You should also have a good idea of what your practice is worth from Chapter 5 and a good understanding of the compensation and deal structure pitfalls from Chapters 6 and 7.

So enter into formal negotiations with a high level of confidence. Now you're ready to make your case that the robustness of your business makes you an attractive candidate to fit into the hospital's strategy.

THE ROLE OF OUTSIDE ADVISORS

Many physicians have told me over the years, "Physicians aren't very good at business." My retort is that people in business make even worse physicians. I have worked with many physicians who are very astute at business. In my experience, the danger is physicians who *think* they are astute when they aren't.

I'll leave it to you decide where you fit in this equation, but remember the old adage in the legal profession that an attorney who represents himself has a fool for a client. This adage has a lesson for physicians as well.

You will need a good healthcare attorney to review the agreements and make sure your interests are protected. Most practices have an attorney they consult on general business matters, but healthcare has its own unique legal issues. I've been in meetings with veteran attorneys whose dismal lack of healthcare experience borders on malpractice when advising their clients on a practice sale. They treat the sale as any other business transaction, often to the detriment of their client.

Don't get your attorney involved too early. Usually you don't need an attorney before you have a formal offer and draft asset purchase and employment agreements for review. Many of the business points of the deal are likely not up for negotiation. Hospitals with experience in buying physician practices and employing physicians generally have a model they follow and are unlikely to vary from it in any major way.

You need to focus your efforts on things that are important to you in the longer term, such as base salary, productivity standards, incentive compensation, and input into management. To objectively evaluate these items, you probably will need a practice consultant.

You may already have a trusted practice consultant you can rely on to help you through the process. Many CPA firms provide excellent consulting services to their clients, and some don't. Most CPAs view themselves as consultants; however, like attorneys, finding one with the specialized expertise you really need isn't always that easy. Here, too, experience is the key component.

There are many excellent independent practice consulting firms as well. If you don't know where to start, ask some of your physician colleagues or check with your local medical society. The hospital may also be able to refer you to an experienced firm.

In my experience, one thing above all that exposes an inexperienced advisor—be it an attorney or consultant—is an almost singular focus on price (i.e., the value of your practice). Inexperienced advisors often do not understand the nuances and perspectives of the parties and seek to show their worth by trying to get a higher price for your practice. While price is important, there are often other, more important considerations.

Avoid practice brokers: Most are simply trying to gain their commission, which is generally a percentage of the sales price. Therefore, they focus solely on price with little or no expertise or understanding of the complex valuation, compensation, and the all-important post-sale issues.

The cost of hiring legal and consulting professionals often comes into play here as well. You get what you pay for, and all advisors aren't created equal. Back in the 1990s, it was fairly common for the acquiring hospital to reimburse the physician at closing for legal and consulting fees. That is uncommon this time around. Don't forget, you are talking about your livelihood here, and it is in your best interest to spend a few thousand dollars to protect yourself and fully understand the implications of what is being proposed.

INITIAL HOSPITAL MEETING

After the valuation of your practice has been completed, there will be a meeting at which the hospital is expected to make its initial offer. View this meeting as a preliminary sales meeting where the hospital is making its sales presentation; your attorney or consultant need not attend. The tone of this meeting will change if advisors are present asking detailed questions. When in doubt, ask the hospital what the agenda for the meeting is and then make your decision.

Make sure this meeting is scheduled at a time when you will not be distracted by the need to get back to work and that your schedule is flexible in case the meeting runs over. Review the meeting agenda in advance and don't be afraid to set out what you expect to be covered (checklists in this chapter and in Chapter 9 may help you).

Sometimes this meeting turns out to be disappointing in its lack of details and substance. There can be many reasons for this. Sometimes the hospital hasn't had adequate time to prepare. Sometimes it is simply trying to gauge your interest or gather additional information about your motivations and plans. For example, a question often asked in the hospital administrative suite is what is motivating a physician to sell. Is he or she interested in retiring early or in slowing down? Is the reason given for wanting to sell the "real" reason, or is there some other hidden agenda that needs to be ferreted out?

Anticipate these questions and be clear at the outset about your needs and desires. Always act in good faith and be honest about your intentions. As noted before, there are no secrets in medical communities.

Before you go into this meeting, you should take some time with your practice consultant to sketch out, at least on a preliminary basis, the major components of an acceptable deal. Emotions have no place here. If you've completed the valuation worksheet in Chapter 5, you should have a ballpark idea of the value of your practice, what level of salary and bonus structure would be acceptable, and what other terms and conditions are important to you. This initial meeting isn't the time to bring these up because you will just be learning the hospital's assumptions.

In negotiation meetings, physicians often wear their emotions on their sleeve and talk too much. The hospital representatives may ask what would be an acceptable price for your practice or acceptable compensation. Play your cards close to the vest. There's no upside in telling the hospital how much you think your practice is worth or what salary you think it should offer at this point.

During this initial meeting, maintain a calm demeanor and listen. A hospital acquiring your practice is, at its core, about creating value through the combination of efforts. Negotiation, therefore, will ultimately center on who claims that value.

Physicians often focus too much on the value of their practice. Generally your compensation is much more important. When hospitals bought practices in the 1990s, they offered physicians large, long-term, guaranteed base salaries. Then they watched physician productivity plummet by an average of 20% to 25%. Hospitals learned their lesson, so don't expect the security of a long-term guaranteed contract. Expect a base salary typically based on prior-year earnings and guaranteed only for a relatively short period, such as one or two years. Expect that meeting productivity standards will be a part of the guarantee.

In general, the value of your practice is not up for a lot of negotiation. The hospital is limited to the value as determined by the independent valuation firm, so negotiation on the valuation usually is limited to areas where underlying assumptions were not correct. Many hospitals won't share the valuation report with you, but some will. It doesn't hurt to ask, as it can provide some insight into the valuation assumptions. Being able to challenge those assumptions may provide some ammunition for future negotiating.

As discussed in Chapter 5, the assumptions made by the appraiser affect the value of your practice and the compensation being offered. Your goal during this initial meeting should be to gather as much information as possible and learn what these assumptions are. It may be possible to have the assumptions reevaluated if they do not fairly reflect the financial performance of the practice, but not at this initial meeting. Gather data, ask questions, and plan to come back later fully armed.

The questions you should ask at this first meeting depend on the level of detail the hospital gets into. Here is a list of some potential questions you should be prepared to ask if the hospital discusses your practice's valuation and proposed compensation, and a brief discussion of each:

1. **What is the projected revenue of the practice over the first few years after acquisition?** The valuation firm likely will base this number on your historical revenue. If your recent historical revenue was lower or higher because of unusual circumstances, ask if those circumstances were considered. Common examples include changes in providers, such as the hiring or departure of an associate physician or midlevel provider; changes in work days for personal reasons, such as illness or injury; or the recent addition of a new ancillary service that may not be fully reflected in last year's income statement. Billing and collection problems

also can have an impact on these assumptions. While you may hesitate to admit your practice has had operational issues, it will ultimately be to your benefit to make sure the revenue reflects the true revenue-producing ability of your practice.

2. **What is the projected revenue growth rate in the practice, and what is it based on?** The valuation firm likely will project future revenue growth based on your practice's historical growth or the regional or national growth trends in your specialty. You should know your practice's historical revenue growth trend and any reasons this growth was less than what you expect in the future. Demonstrating an understanding of your practice's finances can never hurt, and false assumptions can sometimes be changed if supported by concrete data.

3. **What method was used to value the furniture and equipment?** The typical methods used are described in Chapter 4, and in most cases, it doesn't make a lot of difference which method is used. At this stage you are gathering information. Refrain from judgments.

    If the value of your furniture and equipment is significantly different than the estimate you gained from the worksheets in Chapter 4, ask if it would be possible to get an itemized list of furniture and equipment to review for completeness. While many hospitals won't share the complete valuation report, most will provide the furniture and equipment listing and related valuation.

4. **Is value consideration being given for medical records and a trained workforce in place?** As noted in Chapter 5, many hospitals simply will not pay for intangible assets. Some will, but only if the value is supported by a positive value by the income approach. However, both of these positions are changing in some markets based on the supply and demand and other competitive pressures discussed in Chapter 5.

    Here again, the importance of market intelligence cannot be overemphasized. There are very few secrets in most medical communities, and you should speak to peers and colleagues who sold their practices before you and get a feel for what your hospital has done in the past and is currently doing.

Discussions at the initial meeting should also include issues such as what operational changes will take place post-sale. This discussion will supplement your earlier research in choosing a hospital. A desirable hospital partner will have clear answers about post-sale operational issues because it will have experience dealing with these issues in previous acquisitions as well as in practice management.

Don't be put off by nonspecific answers. It is not unusual for hospitals to be examining many potential acquisitions simultaneously, and the final answer as to how these will be integrated is often something driven by timing. What you are looking for is some substance and an indication that these items have been or are being given serious consideration.

Finally, consider with whom you are meeting. The hospital CEO may not be the most well-versed member of hospital management to address some of these issues. Hospitals experienced in practice acquisitions and physician employment will have professional practice management personnel at the meeting. These people are usually more capable of addressing these detail questions.

Timing is an important question you should be prepared to discuss at this initial meeting. There always seems to be a propensity, often driven by both sides, to "get the deal done." This is not always in your best interest. For example, if your bonus is dependent on cash collections, rushing the deal through without providing adequate time for transfer of provider numbers and payor credentialing will likely result in disappointing first-year performance and diminished bonuses.

Over-anxiousness on your part to get the deal done in an unrealistic time frame can also be construed as a sign that your practice is faltering or, even worse, as a sign of negotiating weakness.

Take notes, but it is usually best to refrain from expressing strong opinions. At this stage, the hospital likely will not be presenting formal legal agreements. You should, however, expect the hospital to provide a nonbinding term sheet outlining the major terms of the proposed offer. If one isn't provided, ask that one be sent to you within a short period of time after the meeting.

Ask that the term sheet be specific to your practice and include a detailed description of base salary, productivity standards, and incentive compensation. Ask for an example of how incentive compensation is calculated to help you and your advisors understand what is being proposed.

Try to leave the first meeting with a second meeting scheduled and firm deadlines for the hospital to get back to you with answers to your questions and any additional items it promises to provide as a result of the meeting. Make sure that it provides the information promised enough in advance to allow you to review and react to its written responses.

NEGOTIATING STRATEGY

After the initial meeting, you should have the hospital's initial offer. Now it is time for you to step back for some deliberate consideration and strategizing.

Compare the offer to your initial expectations. If it is significantly different, you may want to work with your practice consultant to break down the differences. Use the Chapter 5 valuation worksheet to raise additional questions.

The answers to the questions you asked in the initial meeting and the comparison to your initial expectations should provide some insight as to how the hospital and its valuation firm arrived at their initial offer. While your practice's value may not be negotiable, understanding and challenging the underlying assumptions can result in a revised offer that may more closely reflect your expectations.

Here is a list of major issues that may need further review and clarification:

Asset value

Compare the asset value offered with your expectation. Review the equipment list and values for completeness. While the valuation method generally isn't negotiable, errors and omissions in the asset list should be updated. In addition, some major items can have values well in excess of the typical valuation methods used (as described in Chapter 5). Examples include ophthalmology and imaging equipment such as ultrasound machines, x-ray equipment, and CT scanners. Do your own Internet research if necessary.

Practice value

If the practice has no intangible value, make sure you understand the assumptions used in the financial projections. Use the worksheet in Chapter 4 to highlight issues for discussion. As noted above, most hospitals will not share the valuation report, but they will answer your questions on issues such as projected revenue growth, overhead growth, and post-sale provider compensation.

Given the recent valuation trends, discussed at the end of Chapter 5, you may want to have your advisor make the case for intangible value regardless of the hospital's valuation. Specific assets you should consider seeking a value for include medical records and a trained workforce in place.

As noted above, the fact that a particular hospital is paying for intangible value often becomes known among the medical staff, so doing some covert intelligence with your peers and colleagues may also be helpful and help bolster your case.

Base salary

Make sure you understand how the base salary offer was determined and what productivity standards, if any, are required to earn that salary. Base salary and the period it is guaranteed, if any, is often negotiable.

Incentive compensation

Be sure you understand the incentive compensation methodology and have been provided with both a written description and a sample calculation. Pay close attention to where the numbers come from and how they relate to your current performance.

Follow-up hospital meetings

There may be other minor issues that need clarification as well. At this point, negotiations generally go back and forth. The hospital may engage its advisors in these discussions. Depending on the nature and importance of the issues, it may be appropriate at this point for your advisors to attend these meetings as well.

Maintain a list or log of negotiating points and keep track of the status of each one. An example of this log is included at the end of this chapter, along with a sample form.

You may wish to include questions from Chapter 9 in your discussions with the hospital (see Chapter 9 checklist).

REACHING A DECISION POINT

The time will come when you realize that what is on the table is about the best you're going to do. You should be able to recognize how well-versed and experienced the hospital is in practice acquisitions by how it handled the negotiations,. Even though you may not have gotten everything you wanted, the insight you gained from the negotiations and the hospital's explanations of various issues should tell you the rest of what you need to know to make your final decision.

Maybe that decision is clear. If it isn't, take some time now to read through Chapter 11: Options Other than Selling. These options (and your willingness to invest the time, effort, and money in pursuing them) may help you come to a final decision.

HOSPITAL PERSPECTIVE

Most hospitals find it exasperating to deal with inexperienced attorneys and consultants. Sometimes advisors take on what I like to call the role of "the unwinder." An unwinder is simply someone who could be acting to protect a vested interest—in this case a long-standing client. Objective advisors will do their best to understand a physician's motivations to sell and help the physician understand if the post-sale results will meet those needs.

I have seen attorneys create unwarranted adversarial situations, and I've seen hospitals simply walk away. At its core, the sale of a practice is a common and straightforward business transaction. There may be many physicians clamoring to sell; as noted in Chapter 4, it is still a buyer's market in most areas. At this late stage of the game (see Chapter 1), the hospital's acquisition policies and valuation models are likely well-established and likely not very negotiable.

At some point, the hospital may lump you in with your inappropriately troublesome attorney and decide purchasing your practice is simply not worth the trouble.

As markets mature and hospitals find themselves with dozens or even hundreds of employed physicians, the less room there will be in negotiating contract language. As any organization grows, so does the need for standardization. So if you are looking at joining a well-established hospital–physician network, you should anticipate contract terms, valuation, and compensation models that are close to non-negotiable.

The best strategy is the deliberate approach described here. Hospitals respect physicians who know their practice and are reasonable in their negotiations. Unreasonable demands and threats to redirect referrals if you don't get what you want are not negotiating strategies; they are soliciting an illegal inducement and will give hospitals another reason to walk away.

TAKEAWAY POINTS FOR CHAPTER 8

1. You will need a healthcare attorney experienced in practice sales to review the agreements and make sure your interests are protected.
2. You also will need an experienced healthcare consultant.
3. Don't get your attorney involved too early. Usually you don't need an attorney until you have a formal offer and draft asset purchase and employment agreements for review.
4. It is in your best interest to spend a few thousand dollars to hire experienced advisors to protect yourself and help you fully understand the implications of what is being proposed.
5. After the valuation of your practice has been completed, there will be a meeting at which the hospital is expected to make its initial offer. Before you go into this meeting, you should take some time with your practice consultant to sketch out, at least on a preliminary basis, the major components of an acceptable deal.
6. Consider pushing for a value that includes medical records and a trained workforce in place. Know what the hospital has offered other physicians in the area.
7. If you are joining a well-established hospital–physician network, you should anticipate contract terms, valuation, and compensation models that are close to non-negotiable.

8. Physicians often focus too much on the value of their practice. Generally your compensation is much more important.

9. The value of your practice is generally not up for a lot of negotiation. The hospital is limited to the value as determined by the independent valuation firm.

10. Many hospitals will not share the valuation report with you, but some will. It doesn't hurt to ask, as it can provide some insight to the valuation assumptions and may provide some ammunition for negotiating later.

11. Your goal during the initial post-valuation meeting should be to gather as much information as possible and learn what the underlying assumptions are. It may be possible to have the assumptions reevaluated if they do not fairly reflect the financial performance of the practice. Gather data, ask questions, and plan to come back later fully armed.

12. Ask that the hospital provide a nonbinding term sheet outlining the major terms of the proposed offer. It should include a detailed description of base salary, productivity standards, and incentive compensation. Ask for an example of how incentive compensation is calculated to help you and your advisors understand what is being proposed.

13. After you have the hospital's initial offer, step back for some deliberate consideration and strategizing. Compare the offer with your initial expectations. If it is significantly different, you may want to work with your practice consultant to break down the differences.

14. Maintain a list or log of negotiating points and keep track of the status of each one.

15. You should be able to recognize—by how the hospital handled the negotiations—how well-versed and experienced it is in practice acquisitions. The insight you gained from the negotiations and the hospital's explanations of various issues should tell you the rest of what you need to know to make your final decision.

16. If the decision isn't clear, read through Chapter 11: Options Other Than Selling. These options and your willingness to invest the time, effort, and money in pursuing them, may aid you in coming to a final decision.

CHECKLIST: THE INITIAL HOSPITAL MEETING

After the valuation of your practice has been completed, there will be a meeting at which the hospital is expected to make its initial offer. Although no checklist can be entirely comprehensive, this checklist covers the many of the steps you should take.

Before the Initial Meeting

Take some time with your practice consultant to sketch out, at least on a preliminary basis, the major components of an acceptable deal:

1. A ballpark idea of the value of your practice. (See Chapter 5 worksheet.)
2. The level of salary and bonus structure that would be acceptable.
3. Other terms and conditions that are important to you.

During the Initial Meeting

Your goal during the initial post-valuation meeting should be to gather as much information as possible.

1. Learn the underlying assumptions the hospital used for its calculations. It may be possible to have the assumptions reevaluated if they do not fairly reflect the financial performance of the practice.
2. Gather data, ask questions, and plan to come back later fully armed.
3. When the hospital discusses your practice valuation and proposed compensation (at this meeting or later), ask these questions if they are not already answered:
   - What is the projected revenue of the practice over the first few years after acquisition?
   - What is the projected revenue growth rate in the practice, and what is it based on?
   - What method was used to value the furniture and equipment?
   - Is value consideration being given for medical records and a trained workforce in place?
   - What operational changes will happen post-sale? (See Chapter 9 checklists.)
   - What is the general, expected timing for purchase? Does it allow adequate time for transfer of provider numbers and payor credentialing?
4. During the meeting or soon afterward, ask that the hospital provide the following:
   - A nonbinding term sheet outlining the major terms of the proposed offer. It should include a detailed description of base salary, productivity standards, and incentive compensation.
   - An example of how incentive compensation is calculated, to aid you and your advisors in understanding what is being proposed.
   - An appointment time for the next meeting.
   - Agreed-on deadlines for further information the hospital will provide to you.

After the Initial Meeting

Once you have the hospital's initial offer, step back for some deliberate consideration and strategizing.

1. Compare the offer with your initial expectations (Chapter 5 worksheet). If it is significantly different, you may want to work with your practice consultant to break down the differences.

2. Maintain a list or log of negotiating points and keep track of the status of each one. (See Sample Negotiating Log.)

3. Review the insights you gained from the meeting and the hospital's explanations of various issues. These should help guide you as you make your final decision to proceed or not.

Sample Negotiating Log

Issue	Equipment value
Description	Doesn't include new furniture purchased this year; hospital indicated they would update value on provision of documentation.
Action/Status	June 3: Provided hospital copies of invoices.
Expected Resolution	Hospital should agree to increase equipment value to reflect the $8,900 cost of these items.

Issue	Base salary
Description	Base salary offered is based on last year's income which was down as a result of billing issues that have been resolved this year.
Action/Status	Provided hospital charge and collection data for the past 18 months to show improvement.
Expected Resolution	Hospital should revise projections and base salary on updated numbers reflecting the current year's trend.

Issue	Incentive compensation
Description	Incentive is based on patient encounters. Need to understand how encounters target was established and how it relates to my practice's historical data.
Action/Status	Hospital is to provide written definition and worksheet showing its calculation of my encounters last year.
Expected Resolution	Encounter target needs to be based on the above calculation and contractual definition needs to match calculation.

Negotiating Log Form

Issue	
Description	
Action/Status	
Expected Resolution	

Issue	
Description	
Action/Status	
Expected Resolution	

CHAPTER 9

Operational and Post-Sale Issues

All marriages are happy. It's the living together afterward that causes all the trouble. RAYMOND HULL

As difficult and time-consuming as it can be to get the deal done, myriad issues can arise after the sale as well. Problems these issues create can be minimized if they are addressed during the sale process, so be sure to include questions from this chapter in your discussions with the hospital.

The biggest issues post-sale usually take place during the transition from independent practice to hospital-owned. In every sale transaction, there is a closing during which everyone signs the agreements, funds change hands, and an effective date is established. The effective date is often the day after closing. Everything from the effective date forward such as billing, personnel, payroll, benefits, accounts payable, and accounting are now legally the responsibility of your new employer, the hospital.

All of these issues should be considered prior to the effective date, and both parties should understand how they will be handled.

TIMING

As noted earlier, often there is a drive in a practice sale to "get the deal done." This is not always in the best interest of either party. This urgency is driven just as often by the physicians as by the hospital. Once you've made the decision to sell and negotiated your best deal, it is understandable that you're ready to get on with it.

The hospital often has the same anxiousness: It has made its decision, too, and often wants to move on. The hospital's business strategy may come into play as well. For example, if the strategy is to renegotiate payor contracts around the broader physician network, the hospital wants that network in place as soon as possible.

The hospital may defer to you on determining the effective date. What an appropriate timeframe is will vary depending on the circumstances. For example, if practice billing is going to be moved on to the hospital's system, more time may be needed for hardware and software installation and staff training than if current systems will remain in place.

The best approach with timing is to establish a reasonable effective date and predicate that date on milestones being met. Checklist 1 at the end of this chapter lists typical critical path items that need to be considered in establishing an effective date. A flexible effective date conditioned on identifiable milestones will serve both parties better than an artificial date that has to be adhered to at all costs.

TRANSITION ISSUES

Transitions are difficult by their nature; mounds of details need to be dealt with. Many of the problems can be minimized with good advance planning and attention to detail. Let's look at some of the major issues and how to minimize their effects.

Provider numbers and payor credentialing

Provider numbers and payor credentialing is often a complex issue. What needs to be done varies significantly depending on the organizational structure of the hospital's ownership, ever-changing regulations, and even varying interpretations of those regulations by fiscal intermediaries.

Hospital administration is generally not well-versed in the detail requirements, so experienced personnel are important. Regardless, it is hard to push bureaucracies; they move at their own pace. Medicare usually isn't as big a potential problem as the commercial payors. Medicare allows retroactive billing, so even if it takes several months to get the paperwork straightened out, the money will eventually come in. This isn't true with most commercial payors.

Sometimes it seems as if commercial payors deliberately drag out the process because they typically don't allow retroactive billing. If your effective date is before everything is completed, the payors know you'll likely continue to see their patients—effectively for free—so there is little incentive for them to cooperate. Rushing the effective date without everything in place plays right into their hands.

If the parties are pushing for an effective date without allowing a minimum of 60 days to complete the provider number and credentialing work (90 or 120 days is often more realistic), the potential losses are huge.

This is also where the structure of your incentive compensation is important. If the hospital insists on forging ahead and billing and collection problems result, you want to make sure your bonus is not based on those collections or profitability because the problems then inevitably affect your income. Even if the resulting billing and collection issues are not your fault and don't directly affect you bonus, hospital management may find itself having to explain unexpected operating losses that may taint your practice's reputation.

Staff issues

Your staff members will be going through a transition also, and they likely will have a lot of questions and concerns about their salaries, benefits, and job security. Their job descriptions and reporting lines may change as well. Small medical practices usually have ripe rumor mills. It is unlikely you'll get to this point without having to address the rumor that you're selling to the hospital.

In an independent physician practice, the staff knows who the ultimate authority is: the physician owners. Once the sale to the hospital is complete, this is often less clear.

While many hospitals have a general hands-off policy on most day-to-day operational issues, many physicians sell their practices to be out from under these responsibilities. That can be a double-edged sword. Conflicts arise and staff members can get caught in the middle between the hospital's practice manager, to whom they technically report, and the physician, who is used to being in charge.

Even if the hospital has a hands-off policy, that doesn't mean nothing changes. While this issue varies depending on the legal structure the hospital uses, it is likely your staff members are now employees of the hospital or one of its affiliated companies and therefore subject to the hospital's personnel policies. Hospitals are subject to employment laws from which most small practices are exempt, such as the Family and Medical Leave Act.

Hospital personnel policies probably are more stringent and formalized. For example, there likely is a formal process that has to be followed before a staff member can be terminated. Staff evaluations are probably more formalized and mandatory. Work rules such as break time and overtime requirements most likely are less flexible.

Most hospitals have salary scales based on job classifications. Progress through these salary scales often is based on years of service. Future staff raises may be subject to these pay scales and the hospital's budgets. Hospitals generally have higher salary scales and more generous employee benefits. These additional costs can affect your overhead and incentive compensation as well.

The process for hiring staff may also become more complex. While it may be a relief to have the hospital source and screen candidates, the hiring process can sometimes seem slow and cumbersome.

Almost assuredly, your staff members will be quite concerned about changes in their benefits. While in most cases, fringe benefits such as health insurance and retirement benefits improve under hospital employment, problems can arise for long-term employees whose years of service provide them with additional vacation and sick days. Hospitals sometimes refuse to grandfather these benefits. Staff may not like these changes, resulting in increased turnover.

Before the effective date, the hospital should schedule a meeting with your staff members to explain the employee manual and answer staff questions about benefits and other changes. Often, hospital personnel policies require a formal staff orientation.

Financial reports

Almost all physician practices use the cash basis of accounting, while hospitals are required by generally accepted accounting principles to report their financial results on the accrual basis. In the simplest terms, here is the difference: To a physician, cash collections equal revenue. To a hospital, revenue is what it *expects* to collect from gross charges, so it must be estimated.

Accounting is simply dividing the financial results of a business into artificial periods such as months, quarters, and years. Over the life of any business, cash and accrual accounting will ultimately lead to the same financial results. Problems arise when hospitals try to get physicians to understand accrual accounting, and this is especially true during the early stages of employment when the lack of historical collection data can make accurately estimating accrual basis revenue impossible.

While many hospitals have learned this lesson and prepare separate financial reports for their employed physicians on a cash basis, the larger the hospital's employed physician group becomes, the more likely they will insist on using accrual basis.

If all or part of your compensation is based on revenue, such as under a profit-based incentive or the virtual private practice models discussed in Chapter 6, make sure you understand how the estimate of accrual basis revenue is made and assure it is reasonably accurate.

Vendor payments

After the effective date, all your practice's bills—utilities, rent, telephone, and supplies—become the responsibility of the hospital. As a practical matter, it is impossible to get all your vendor accounts transferred into the hospital's name on the effective date. While this usually isn't a major issue, it does mean that somebody has to be on top of these details to make sure the bills get paid on a timely basis and that ultimately the funds get accounted for properly.

Generally, the hospital will handle the payments after the effective date. In cases where invoices include both pre- and post-sale charges, a list of payments is generally maintained along with an allocation of what is the practice's responsibility and what is the hospital's responsibility. Generally, the totals are reconciled after 60 to 90 days, and any amounts due-to/due-from are settled and paid.

HOSPITAL PERSPECTIVE

Problems with post-sale issues tend to arise with inexperienced hospitals; hospitals that have experience have systems and procedures in place to address these issues.

Inexperienced hospitals often default to doing things through existing hospital systems and bureaucracy. If the hospital with which you have chosen to affiliate lacks experience, it is incumbent on you and your advisors to carefully work through the issues discussed in this chapter in advance. Inflexibility and inexperience are a bad combination. These issues can be critical to getting the relationship off to a good start, and failure to adequately deal with them may even reach the level of causing you to revisit your decision.

TAKEAWAY POINTS FOR CHAPTER 9

1. Myriad issues can arise after the sale, and these can be minimized if they are addressed during the sale process.
2. There often is a drive in a practice sale to "get the deal done." This is not always in the best interest of either party.
3. A flexible effective date conditioned on identifiable milestones will serve both parties better than an artificial date that has to be adhered to at all costs.
4. If the parties are pushing for an effective date without allowing a minimum of 60 days—and 90 or 120 days is often more realistic—to complete the provider number and credentialing work, the potential losses are huge.
5. Your staff members will be going through a transition also, and probably have a lot of questions and concerns about their salaries, benefits, and job security.
6. Your staff members are now employees of the hospital or one of its affiliated companies and probably are subject to the hospital's personnel policies.
7. Before the effective date, the hospital should schedule a meeting with your staff to explain its employee manual and answer staff questions about benefits and other changes.
8. Problems always arise when hospitals try to get physicians to understand accrual accounting. Most hospitals have learned this lesson and prepare separate

financial reports for their employed physicians on a cash basis, but you should ask just to make sure.

9. Somebody has to be on top of the detail of vendor payments to make sure the bills get paid on a timely basis and that ultimately the funds get accounted for properly.

10. These issues can be critical to getting the relationship off to a good start, and failure to adequately deal with them may even reach the level of causing you to revisit your decision.

Checklist 1: Critical Path Items in Establishing an Effective Date

❏ Payor credentialing
- Medicare number transfers
- Medicaid
- Commercial payors

❏ Personnel
- Staff informational meetings

❏ Staff orientation and/or policy manual review
- Benefit enrollment
- Payroll

❏ Billing system
- Hardware, software, and data line installation
- Demographic data transfer
- Staff training
- Revisions to financial policies

❏ Accounts payable
- Approval process
- Payment policies and procedures
- Vendor account transfers
- Pre- and post-sale invoice reconciliation plan

❏ Malpractice
- Tail premium if changing carriers
- Changes in coverage
- Other

Checklist 2: Operational/Staff Issues to Discuss with the Hospital

❏ How and by whom will vendor payments be handled during the first transitional months?

❏ Can the hospital's financial reports be generated on a cash basis for physicians?

❏ Does the hospital have a "hands-off" or an "involved" policy for day-to-day operational issues concerning your staff? Does that align with your preference?

❏ How will your staff be informed about salaries, benefits, and job security? Will the hospital schedule a meeting with your staff to explain its employee manual and answer staff questions about benefits and other changes?

❏ How will staff job descriptions and reporting lines change?

❏ How will benefits such as health insurance and retirement benefits improve or change under hospital employment? Problems can arise for long-term employees who have years of service that provide them with additional vacation and sick days. Does the hospital grandfather these benefits?

❏ Since your staff will likely be subject to the hospital's personnel policies, are those policies more stringent and formalized? What process must be followed before a staff member can be terminated? How are staff evaluations handled? What are the work rules for things such as break time and overtime?

❏ Hospitals generally have higher salary scales for staff and more generous employee benefits; how will these additional costs affect your overhead and incentive compensation?

❏ What is the hospital's process for hiring staff?

CHAPTER 10

Making It Work

I t is a different time and a different place, but we've been down this road before. The fits and starts of the past 15 to 20 years have given way to hospital–physician networks that, unlike those of the 1990s, absolutely and positively need to work over the long term. Unfortunately, the mistakes of the 1990s are being repeated in many markets. As a result, the sustainability of these networks, as discussed in Chapter 1, is coming into question as the level of losses are reaching what could be unsustainable levels.

The option for physicians to join hospital networks, decide they don't like the arrangement, and go back out into private practice is a much more daunting proposition today than it was a decade or two ago. My company examines dozens of independent physician-owned medical practices each year, and a huge percentage of them have physician owners earning below—in many cases substantially below—the median income for their specialty. As discussed in Chapter 2, one reason for this is biases in the survey data.

Conversely, as losses from these networks mount, the option for hospitals to decide that they can simply divest themselves of their physician practices is equally specious.

Healthcare is changing. Healthcare needs to change. This was true with or without health reform and will continue to be true. The current payment mechanisms based on volume are expected to evolve to be based more on outcomes, quality, coordination of care, and wellness. Indeed, the repeal of the SGR formula for Medicare payment discussed in Chapter 2 put in place a pathway for Medicare payment to be increased based on these factors. Hospitals and physicians must work together to figure out how to make the system work under these new structures.

In many ways, what happens as physicians sell their practices to hospitals is analogous to a shotgun wedding in which both parties rush down the aisle without sufficient time to plan their life together. And that is where the trouble begins. The reality sets in soon afterward that what has been created is an unmanageable monster.

As physicians settle into ongoing employment relationships with hospital systems, new ways of doing business will be necessary if both sides wish to avoid the train wreck that happened last time around. How will the relationships and organizations need to evolve? What red flags loom? We are seeing some of them now: huge financial losses, mismanagement, and even physicians returning to private practice. The rules will have to change, and fresh thinking will be needed with both physicians and hospitals adjusting to avoid a repeat of history. After the honeymoon is over, how do the two partners work together to ensure a successful evolution of a sustainable relationship?

THEY DON'T KNOW WHAT THEY DON'T KNOW

Perhaps the most important aspect that has to change is that hospitals have to recognize they don't know what they don't know.

Hospital systems usually employ many bright, highly educated people who, while they may be excellent stewards of hospital sustainability and success, have no real understanding of the business of physician practice. Running a successful hospital is dramatically different than running a successful physician organization. The latter comprises previously independent practices, and it takes great skill (and care) for small cottage industries to successfully evolve to be part of larger organizations.

The old adage that managing physicians is like herding cats is largely accurate, but it is no excuse for lack of engagement. Running a physician enterprise is a difficult task that needs to be molded into the overall business of providing healthcare for the community the system serves. Failing to acknowledge the cultural and structural differences and trying to mold the physician network into a hospital-centric system full of silos, mini-empires, politics, and bureaucratic policies is a recipe for failure.

GOVERNANCE AND LEADERSHIP

In Chapter 4, I cited investment in technology and experienced practice management executives as predictors of success in physician networks. But money coupled with lip service will not produce success. Do actions follow the words?

In the 1990s, hospitals sold physicians on the idea of employment by promising: "We'll take care of the business side; you just practice medicine." This time around, as noted in Chapter 7, successful models often tout how the full engagement of physicians in governance of the organization will assure its success. While ultimately, everybody understands that "he who has the gold makes the rules," the theorem postulated is that significant control over both day-to-day operations and longer-term strategic planning needs to be delegated to physician-led boards and operating councils. These entities, in partnership with senior hospital management, determine the direction of the organization.

While I support these strategies, in the real world they are often ineffective. Unfortunately, in many situations, physician governance is relegated to nothing more than keeping the physicians informed and on board with a hospital-centric strategy.

As discussed in Chapter 1, while engaging physicians in governance is almost universally touted as a key tenet of the success of an integrated network, the harsh reality is that this "governance," generally because of legal restrictions, usually comes with little or no authority. It often is no more than a feeble and transparent attempt to co-opt physician leadership to the hospital side in economic discussions and ultimately provide cover for a restructuring of physician compensation in order to reduce losses.

Hospitals have been giving lip service to the idea of having physicians in leadership roles for decades. While that has changed in many markets and physicians have become more willing to step up and participate, the results are often less than satisfactory. Whether doctors should be in leadership positions to the exclusion of delivering patient care is another question, however. Doctors who become full-time administrators often are viewed by their peers as "suits" and often lose credibility and the respect of their colleagues.

The reporting line for senior leadership of the physician enterprise (i.e., the practice administrator or executive director) is often a good indicator of the level of respect that person and the physician enterprise have within the hospital system. Reporting to a second- or third-level (below the CEO) manager, regardless of title, often relegates physician network leadership to a subservient role in decision making and strategic planning. This raises legitimate questions about how important the physician enterprise truly is in the grand scheme of things.

A reasonable degree of structure is necessary, but too many layers of bureaucracy between doctors and top management will drive a wedge between the partners. Successful organizations hire the most qualified, most experienced practice executives they can find and have them report to the highest level of management in the system (often the CEO). To do otherwise sends a message to physicians that they are not important to the organization.

Similarly, what message does it send to the physicians if the senior leadership of the health system delegates participation in governance of the physician enterprise to lower level managers? The importance, and perhaps even the relevance, of this governing body is neutralized without the participation and full engagement of senior hospital management.

The person who signs physician employment agreements for the hospital should be in a seat at the governance table. When he or she is not there, decisions are made without all of the facts, and top-level administration becomes insulated from what's going on at the practice level. Then, when something goes wrong, they complain that they were "in the dark."

ADDRESS RED FLAGS UP FRONT

My company is routinely called in to restructure hospital/physician networks that are on the brink of implosion. While financial results are usually cited as the motivation for the restructuring, almost always the seeds of the problem were sown in the unwillingness to address difficult issues up front. It is almost like a marriage doomed before the wedding because the parties, while acknowledging their differences, believe they can change each other.

Ignoring red flags and failing to address critical issues out of fear of losing the deal can be worse than walking away. Recently, we helped a modestly sized rural hospital structure an acquisition of a three-physician specialty group. The specialists were the only such group in the area and an important part of healthcare in the community. Dr. Watson (not his real name) was the youngest member of the group. After two years of trying to establish his practice, the two senior doctors decided to make him a partner even though his productivity was still 30% below theirs.

When the practice approached the hospital about employment, the executive in charge put together an offer that supplemented Watson's income for one year to allow him to continue to build his practice. When presented with the generous contract, Watson unabashedly stated that if his salary went down at the end of the year, he would be asking the hospital why it hadn't been successful in building his practice!

The group was insistent in retaining Watson and pushed the hospital into a position of agreeing to a losing strategy. As noted in Chapter 2, the belief that hospital employment will solve these types of intra-group issues is not a reason to sell. Sometimes failure can be predicted with a high degree of accuracy. Rather than address the underlying issues, the hospital, against our advice, chose to ignore it, and the deal was signed anyway.

While the physicians felt they had "won" a major negotiating point, their victory was hollow. Watson's inability to build a practice (to say nothing about his attitude) predictably didn't resolve itself, and the outcome was ultimately worse for both sides. The hospital wasted precious resources in artificially supporting what was predestined to be a losing battle, and the two senior partners ended up working longer hours and taking 50% more call to pick up the volume left behind when the disgruntled younger physician departed. Everybody was unhappy. The short-term gain wasn't worth the long-term loss. The result was wholly predictable, and both sides would have been better off addressing it up front.

A hospital's fear of losing the deal often subsumes common sense. Ego prevails, and the result is lost opportunities and setbacks in building toward the long-term goals of both sides. When a friend of mine once lamented, "What was I thinking?" after his divorce was finalized, he was referring to the marriage, not the divorce.

Monitoring performance and holding physicians accountable is critical, and successful hospital networks recognize this fact. Hospital executives are not typically good at making tough decisions related to the medical staff. They've been on the receiving end of the wrath of unhappy doctors often enough that they've learned it's easier (not to mention job-preserving) to acquiesce rather than put up a fight.

For example, Dr. Smith refuses to take weekend call and flirts with the nurses a little. What is a hospital administrator to do? Smith is a big producer and patients love him. Maybe it's best just to look the other way. Wrong. Taking this approach is the marital equivalent of pretending not to know your spouse is having an affair because you like driving a Lexus and living in an upscale neighborhood.

Employed physicians should expect to be held accountable for their end of the partnership, and this is where physician leadership comes into the equation. This means—in addition to being competent and delivering quality medical care—showing up on time when they're scheduled to work, treating support staff with respect, abiding by policies and procedures, representing the organization in a professional manner, and generally working as part of a team.

From time to time, difficult decisions have to be made. Both physician leaders and hospital administrators have to be willing to deal with a doctor who has become a liability. They have to ask themselves what it's costing to keep that doctor on board. What message is it sending to other physicians and to the rest of the staff? Sometimes, an organization grows and thrives by subtraction.

OVER-RELIANCE ON HOSPITAL SYSTEMS AND STAFF

Too often, the thought process of a hospital executive getting into practice acquisition goes something like this: "We have a computer system and people already on board to handle physician billing and accounting. And we have an experienced team in HR. And Jane over in marketing used to work in a big clinic . . . she'd probably jump at the chance to manage a few practices if we gave her a raise. This is great. We're going to save a bundle on overhead and make these new ventures really profitable!"

This is what I call magical thinking: I need for it to be true, so it must be true. One newly formed hospital/physician network our company put together in the Midwest needed to hire a practice manager for one of its offices. Following protocol, the physicians put the job request in with the hospital HR department. Weeks into the process, the doctors in the group couldn't understand why they weren't seeing any candidates. A quick investigation revealed the problem.

The job description developed by the hospital HR department called for someone with an MBA, when someone with a high school diploma and "in the trenches" experience would have been a better candidate. The online job posting linked to the hospital's Web site and a hospital employment application. That application asked such "relevant" questions as "What is your experience working in the ICU?" Many practice manager candidates are leery of working for a hospital anyway, and, in this case, the HR department confirmed their worst suspicions.

Using hospital resources may be fine, but they have to be managed. Adhering to hospital processes without taking the time to rework an employment application or discuss the qualifications for a position is all too typical in large organizations. Using the hospital's HR department may work, but only if physicians or practice managers get involved on the front end to make sure the department's recruiters have a clear understanding that a medical practice is not a small hospital.

On the positive side, hospital HR departments can also be an asset. Turnover is a problem in many small medical practices because they find it economically difficult to offer top pay and benefits. Busy physicians and practice managers are not adept at interviewing candidates and often accept a "warm body" without requisite screening and reference checks. Hospital HR departments often excel at these tasks.

The same issues arise in other hospital support areas. Hospital billing departments generally lack any knowledge or experience in physician billing. Using them to create a central billing office for the physician practices almost always ends in disaster. The hospital finance and accounting department may be full of well-trained CPAs, but they don't utilize or understand the cash basis accounting under which 95% of physician practices historically operate.

As noted in Chapter 4, if hospitals intend to be successful this time around with practice acquisition, they absolutely must invest in an experienced management team and in systems that are designed for medical practices. But even that won't necessarily assure success.

PROFITS, LOSSES, AND PHYSICIAN COMPENSATION

Hospitals that seek to manage physician practices to a breakeven level or to evaluate their performance solely on financial performance perhaps should not be in the business of employing physicians.

In the 1990s, hospitals unceremoniously terminated physician employment agreements when practice losses became the target of bond rating agencies threatening to lower ratings or when a health system's stock prices declined. Health system executives are slowly coming to terms with the fact that physician groups, as distinct departments within the organization, are not likely to be profitable. The paradigm shift that must occur is away from physician as revenue producer to physician as an integral component of delivering quality care and achieving good clinical outcomes.

Some advocate that employed physicians should break even under hospital employment because they did so before selling. This assertion shows a lack of understanding of the economics of small physician practices (or any small business for that matter). The reality is that, absent borrowing to pay owner salaries, any small business "breaks even" because the owner's compensation amounts to what is left after all the bills are paid. I see practices that break even all the time, but in some cases the physicians are earning less than half the median income for their specialty.

The failed economics of private practice is the reality driving the employment of physicians in the first place, so breaking even is and will remain an elusive goal in most markets.

Successful organizations separate controllable versus noncontrollable components and manage to acceptable levels of loss. Some of the controllable factors include:

- Making sure physicians understand the importance of time management, proper scheduling, standardized procedures, and leveraging the EHR to mine data and track productivity and clinical outcomes;
- Creating bullet-proof charge capture systems; and
- Instituting world-class billing and follow-up.

And because dealing in nickels (the $70 office visit) versus dollars (the $2,500 CT scan) requires such a huge shift in thinking, hospital systems that learned from the mistakes of the 1990s know that practices must have their own billing systems. To rely on a hospital-based system is to die a slow, painful financial death.

High-performing hospital/physician networks are also moving away from over-reliance on physician compensation surveys and rules of thumb for what physicians are "normally paid."

The law of supply and demand can't be repealed. We are in the midst of an acute shortage of physicians in primary care and many specialties—a fact that's not likely to change anytime soon. The majority of doctors coming out of residency are saddled with huge debt and are looking for the best deal possible. Hospitals need to be aggressive to attract the best candidates.

One analogy I use to help hospital executives understand how hiring physicians in a competitive market is changing is to have them imagine hiring a new CFO. They would pay what is required to attract the right person with the qualifications and experience necessary to do the job that needs to be done. They might have to pay the CFO a little more than he or she earned in his or her last job. Losing a qualified candidate over a few thousand dollars will almost always come back to haunt the CEO.

While legal considerations with respect to fair market value and commercially reasonable compensation need to be considered, these can be used as an excuse to suppress compensation as opposed to being legitimate legal concerns. However, this is becoming less common because, as discussed in Chapter 6, the compensation expressed by these surveys tends to be high.

TAKEAWAY POINTS FOR CHAPTER 10

1. The option for physicians to join hospital networks, decide they don't like the arrangement, and go back into private practice is a much more daunting proposition today than it was a decade or two ago. The option for hospitals to decide, as losses from these networks mount, that they can simply divest themselves of their physician practices is equally specious.

2. Current payment mechanisms based on volume are expected to evolve to be based more on outcomes, quality, coordination of care, and wellness. Hospital and physicians will need to work together to figure out how to make the system work under these new structures.

3. Hospitals must recognize that they don't know what they don't know. While they usually employ many bright, highly educated people, they often have no real understanding of the business of physician practice.

4. Successful models include the full engagement of physicians in governance of the organization.

5. The reporting line for senior leadership of the physician enterprise (i.e., the practice administrator or executive director) is often a good indicator of the level of respect both that person and the physician enterprise have within the hospital system.

6. The person who signs physician employment agreements for the hospital should be in a seat at the governance table.

7. Almost always, the seeds of problems are sown in the unwillingness to address difficult issues up front. Ignoring red flags and failing to address critical issues out of fear of losing the deal can be worse than walking away.

8. If hospitals intend to be successful this time around with practice acquisition, they absolutely must invest in an experienced management team and in systems that are designed for medical practices. Over-reliance on hospital systems and staff usually fails.

9. Hospitals that seek to manage physician practices to a break-even level or to evaluate their performance solely on financial performance perhaps should not be in the business of employing physicians. Successful organizations separate controllable versus noncontrollable components and manage to acceptable levels of loss.

CHAPTER 11

Options Other Than Selling

Selling your practice is a big decision that likely will impact the rest of your professional career. You may have endured a lengthy process and protracted negotiations and still have some nagging doubts. Are these real or just last-minute jitters?

Go back and review Chapter 2 and the reasons you originally decided to explore selling. Are these reasons still valid? Will the proposed deal likely solve these problems and meet your needs?

Make a list of your concerns with the proposed sale. Are the reasons quantitative—that is, are they based on the financial terms of the deal such as salary and practice value? Or are they qualitative—that is, based on concerns about your chosen hospital partner? Qualitative issues usually are much more important than quantitative ones when it comes to long-term satisfaction.

You may decide that remaining independent is the best course of action, and if you've followed the steps in Chapter 3, you should have a good objective assessment of your practice.

This chapter is about other options or what you may want to do differently in the future.

INTERMEDIATE OPTIONS

In some cases, the fit doesn't seem quite right for various reasons. In many cases, the parties can explore what I call "intermediate models" in an effort to overcome reluctance or differences of opinion on one side or both to an outright sale. For example, you might find after taking an honest assessment of your practice's strengths that the hospital's offer simply isn't adequate, or the hospital may have a reluctance to invest in acquiring physician assets.

Intermediate options include:
- Practice lease;
- Physician enterprise model (PEM); and
- Management services organization (MSO).

Practice lease

A practice lease generally substitutes a lease agreement for the asset purchase agreement. The lease includes the practice's tangible assets and often the intangible assets as well. Typically the hospital leases the practice from you and then contracts with you to provide physician services to the practice's patients for the term of the lease.

This agreement, often referred to as a professional services agreement, functions much like an employment agreement. You agree to provide services to the practice's patients for agreed-upon compensation. The compensation structure typically includes base salary, incentive compensation, and quality incentives as described in Chapter 6. Usually the hospital will take over the management of the practice and employ your staff in the same manner as if you had sold your practice.

Leasing your practice can have some distinct benefits. The principal benefit is that it isn't permanent, so it may be easier to test the waters. A lease will typically have a finite term, often two or three years, so both sides have a date to work toward. At that point, it can be much easier to get out if things aren't working.

Leases can have an option to purchase at a later date, although it would still be subject to an independent valuation at that time. After a year or two, you may find that working for the hospital is going just fine, and price may be less important.

Not all hospitals are willing to offer a practice lease, and don't expect a financial windfall on the lease payments. A lease is basically a payment for the right to use the underlying assets for a finite period of time, so the aggregate lease payments are going to be less than an outright sale because, after the lease term, you will still own the assets.

A weakness in leasing your practice is that you typically cannot be part of the hospital's collective negotiation of payor contracts because technically you are not an employee of the hospital.

Physician enterprise model

Another intermediate model that is a variant of the practice lease is the physician enterprise model (PEM). Again, there are many variations, but under the typical PEM, your practice staff and operations largely remain intact. Your nonprovider employees remain employees of your existing practice entity, which remains in existence, and the hospital "leases" these services for an agreed-upon monthly fee to cover the operating overhead. The monthly fee generally is set in advance based on projected operating overhead, and is often subject to an independent fair market value review.

The providers—typically both physicians and midlevel providers—become employees of the PEM, which usually is a separate entity wholly owned by the hospital. The

PEM compensates the providers based on pre-established contractual terms very similar to what they would have been if you had sold your practice. Here too, the compensation structure typically includes base salary, incentive compensation, and quality incentives as described in Chapter 6.

The biggest difference between a PEM and a practice lease is that under the PEM, you do become an employee of the hospital so you can participate in the hospital's collective negotiation of payor contracts. This potential advantage comes with an offsetting disadvantage though, because usually this means that your billing and collection functions will become part of the hospital's physician billing office, although that is not always the case.

Under a PEM, theoretically, you would be able to easily reestablish private practice at the expiration of the agreement. However, significant barriers will exist at that point.

Once you become an employee of the hospital, your existing A/R, which is generally retained, collected, and distributed as income to the existing owners of your practice, is gone—as are your payor contracts, provider numbers, and (usually) your billing and collection functions. So while your nonbilling staff may still be in place, there are financial implications to restoring independent operations—the largest of which is paying overhead costs and provider salaries while you reestablish billing collection and payor contracts and ramp-up the collections of your "new" A/R to a level that will cover the ongoing overhead. This usually requires a line of credit or other borrowing.

So while the PEM may seem like it allows a simple return to private practice if the relationship doesn't pan out, in reality it has more barriers than a practice lease. However, the PEM does offer some distinct advantages, including:

- Your practice entity, as well as most of your staff and management infrastructure, remains in place with the overhead costs covered by the PEM.
- You access the collective negotiating power and potentially higher payor contract rates of the hospital.
- It generally results in an increase in physician compensation.

In general, the PEM can provide a fair degree of autonomy that might otherwise be lost in an outright sale of your practice.

Management services organization

A management services organization (MSO) is another intermediate model. It simply means contracting with the hospital for the management of your practice by its practice management department. This model is, in many ways, the converse of the PEM.

Many hospitals offer practice management services to physicians using the same infrastructure they created to support the hospital's employed physicians. These services often are available on a fee basis, and physicians can often choose from a menu of services such as billing and collections, HR (including employment of staff), and other practice management services.

A hospital can't legally provide these services for less than fair market value, but this arrangement often can offer independent practices a higher level of practice management expertise, often for the same or slightly higher cost than their current overhead.

A weakness of an MSO is that it cannot collectively negotiate payor contracts for independent groups. But an MSO can take away a majority of the day-to-day management burden and afford you the opportunity to try out the hospital's ability to manage your practice without taking the full step of selling.

The main difference between a practice lease or PEM and an MSO is in the area of compensation:

- In a lease or PEM, the physician compensation is based on a compensation plan, very similar to that under an employment model but coupled with a payment for the lease of the practice assets.
- In an MSO arrangement, the physician turns over management to the hospital, but physician compensation is what is left after payment of the management fee.

Advantages and disadvantages

Intermediate models vary widely, and assessing the advantages and disadvantages in your specific situation can be confusing. Figure 1 summarizes the typical differences among these intermediate models and full employment.

TAKE YOUR PRACTICE TO THE NEXT LEVEL

You may have been happy and successful before the hospital came to call. If that's the case and the hospital's offer simply didn't meet your needs, you might believe that staying independent isn't such a daunting proposition after all.

If you approached the hospital or welcomed its advances because you were frustrated for some or all of the reasons mentioned in Chapter 2, then having the deal fall apart may leave you with a level of dread. If that's the case, go back and reread Chapter 3 on preparing your practice for sale. Take the information and insight you've gained by going through the sales process and use it to chart a different course. (See Checklist 1 at the end of this chapter.)

	Payor Contracting and Billing	Providers Employed by	Staff Employed by	Practice Assets Owned by
Sale	Hospital	Hospital	Hospital	Hospital
Lease	Practice or Hospital	Hospital	Hospital	Practice
PEM	Hospital	Hospital	Practice	Practice
MSO	Practice	Practice	Hospital	Practice

FIGURE 1. Summary of Differences Among Intermediate Models and Full Employment

For better or worse, your practice is a small business. Having a medical license and hanging out your shingle aren't enough anymore. What did you learn about your practice's finances (Chapter 3) that you can improve? Why was your valuation (Chapter 5) less than you had expected? What is your strategic plan? What can you do to improve the situation and either make your practice a better candidate for sale in the future or make it thrive without the need to sell?

Based on 25-plus years working with physician practices, I have found that they stagnate for the following reasons:

1. Aging providers who get comfortable with below-average income levels.
2. An entrenched practice manager (sometimes a spouse) whose skills haven't evolved with the needs of the modern-day practice.
3. An unwillingness to invest in experienced management and billing personnel.
4. An aging patient base, changing demographics in the practice's service area, and deteriorating payor mix.
5. Fear of taking risks in practice expansion through additional physicians, midlevel providers, or ancillary services.
6. Bad experiences with former physician partners, associate physicians, or midlevel providers.
7. Lack of a business plan or strategy to address such things as service niches, ancillary services, mergers, and satellite offices.
8. Poor payor contract rates and lack of data, expertise, and willingness to negotiate better rates, coupled with an unwillingness to terminate marginal contracts.

In a group practice, I would add the following reasons:

1. Behavioral issues or personality clashes with one or more of the physicians.
2. A compensation plan that does not properly incentivize behavior.

If you find one or more of these things prevalent in your practice, the decision is clear: You can continue down your current path or make some hard decisions.

The biggest barrier to change is always the effort required to break habits and take risks. These may include incurring debt to invest in ancillary services or technology, recruiting new physician associates or midlevel providers, hiring a highly qualified (and highly paid) professional manager, or becoming more creative and proactive about promoting your practice.

If you go this route, consider engaging an outside consultant to work with your group to:

- Develop a comprehensive strategic plan;
- Take the emotion out of these decisions and keep you pointed in the right direction;
- Follow through to make the changes needed to improve operations; and
- Monitor progress and keep you focused on results.

MERGE WITH AN EXISTING LARGER GROUP

Many solo practitioners and small groups automatically shun the idea of joining an existing large group practice. This is often based on a bad experience earlier in their career.

Group practice today is much different that it was 10 or 20 years ago. Many long-standing "legacy" groups—groups that were established decades ago—are no longer in business. They became victims of the practice management companies that failed in the 1990s (Chapter 4) or imploded under the weight of their own bureaucracy and management overhead. Those that still exist have been through major restructuring in order to survive.

Many areas of the country have larger group practices that have been created in the past 10 years. These groups are often progressive and successful, with income levels well above national standards. They tend to operate on a model that allows a large degree of physician autonomy, avoids bloated management overhead, and employs aggressive ancillary and payor contracting strategies.

If you've been through the sales process with the hospital, you have already gained valuable knowledge about your business. Don't be scared off by past reputations or ancient history with a larger group—initiate discussions and go through the process to see if you find a better fit.

Some experts believe that in the coming "new world" of value-based payment and population health management, the independent multispecialty group may be the best model. The process of merging your practice with an existing group is, in many ways, quite different than selling to a hospital, but there are similarities as well. You will be asked to provide financial data on your practice, and you should expect the other practice to provide the same data to you.

Just as income was a key component in selling your practice to a hospital, the physicians' incomes are the key component in deciding whether to join the group. Compare their income to yours and to the MGMA benchmarks you reviewed in Chapter 3. Obviously, you are looking for their incomes to be materially higher than yours because, ultimately, their incomes represent your potential income post-merger.

Have your CPA or practice consultant review the financial information the group provides if it seems too overwhelming to do yourself. If the physicians' incomes are higher, you will want to understand why. Do they work more hours? See more patients? Offer more ancillary services?

Other questions you should examine include the following:

1. How does their overhead compare to yours in terms of dollars and percentage?
2. What will happen to your overhead when you join them?
3. Will your costs actually go up because they have higher staff salaries and benefit costs?
4. Will your office be consolidated into one of their locations?

The biggest potential prize in joining a large group is often in the payor contracts. It is unlikely the group will share specific information with you on its payor contracts before completion of the merger, because doing so may constitute illegal price fixing. Ask questions about the group's contracting expertise and abilities. The success of the group's contracts should be evident by looking at the physicians' income levels.

Existing groups never purchase goodwill. Other physicians don't want to invest in your goodwill any more than you would want to invest in theirs. It is likely the group will have a streamlined valuation process and simply offer to purchase your assets. If you went through the process with the hospital, you will have another reference point to determine the reasonableness of the group's offer.

Larger groups also generally have a predefined merger model that is probably not negotiable. Previous mergers were likely carried out under this same model, and varying the model is usually not an option because the precedent has already been set.

You will generally be asked to sign an asset purchase agreement, employment agreement, and buy-sell (shareholders) agreement.

The employment agreement is similar in many ways to the hospital employment agreement discussed in Chapter 6. The most significant difference will be in the compensation sections. Just as in selling to a hospital, the most important aspect is your compensation and bonus structure post-merger. Physician groups generally do not have guaranteed salaries and incentive compensation or bonus plans. Existing group practices have a predetermined method of compensating physician owners, often referred to as a compensation (or income distribution) plan.

The distinction is important but probably not surprising: There are no shareholder guarantees in a group practice any more than there are in a solo practice or small group. Shareholder income is determined by the financial performance of the group.

The complexity of a group's compensation plan often increases with the size of the group. Multispecialty group compensation plans tend to be complex. The group should provide you with a pro forma financial projection of how your practice would fit into the group's existing compensation plan and give you a fairly accurate estimate of what your income would be post-merger.

You should generally expect to come in as an equal owner in the group. Some larger groups, especially those with significant earnings streams coming from ancillary services, may not be willing to offer a newly merged physician a full share of those ancillary profits initially. This may be reasonable, depending on your specialty and the types of ancillaries involved.

Employment agreements with larger group practices generally include a restrictive covenant. While it may seem counterintuitive, you want the group to have one, and you should shy away from any group that doesn't. A physician group is not really a group without some glue holding the physicians together. If people can leave at any time whenever a decision doesn't go their way, the group isn't sustainable. I have seen group practices collapse in short order absent a restrictive covenant.

The buy-sell (or shareholders) agreement is an agreement among all of the partners and dictates how physicians join (buy) and leave (sell) ownership in the practice. Generally the stock buyout will be a share of the value of the assets of the group.

Be wary of buy-sell agreements that provide for excessive buyout payments, deferred compensation, and other provisions for payments to physicians no longer practicing. While a huge golden parachute may sound attractive, the money has to come out of the work of those physicians still in practice.

Large buyout obligations are another reason group practices collapse because, at some point, it is easier to liquidate the group than continue to satisfy huge trailing obligations to physicians who have retired or otherwise left the group.

Some business models for group practices out there have a high probability of problems. Stay away from a group where everyone is not an equal shareholder with an equal vote in the affairs of the group. Group practices owned or controlled by one physician or even a small group of "insider" physicians are generally not sustainable.

Also avoid groups with physician incomes lower than yours. Low incomes in large groups are often caused by bloated overhead, entrenched management, unproductive physicians, substandard billing and collections, and marginal payor contracts.

Out of necessity, large groups have a governance structure that usually consists of a board of directors elected by the shareholders to run the group. The board generally is required to consult the shareholders before making major decisions such as borrowing money in excess of a certain dollar amount, making major capital expenditures, hiring additional physicians, merging with other practices, terminating physicians, changing the compensation plan, and selling the group. These major decisions are often subject to supermajority votes of the shareholders.

Shareholder meetings generally must be held at least once a year, at which time the board of directors is elected. Quarterly meetings are common. Many physicians feel disenfranchised in larger groups because participation in governance is limited to board members. Other physicians may be relieved at not having to be involved in the day-to-day decision making.

Depending on the size of the group, the board may also have standing committees that meet separately and report to the board on issues such as finance, managed care contracting, and compensation. Committee membership is often filled by non-board members, so if participating in the governance of the group is important to you, you will want to ask about these opportunities.

MERGE WITH LIKE-MINDED COLLEAGUES

Becoming larger is one of the classic business strategies used to survive in a changing marketplace. A merger is like a marriage—smaller practices pool their resources for a more effective operation—and all successful marriages require compromises.

Many physicians show a surprising reluctance toward joining a larger group or merging their practices. There are many reasons for this, including previous failed attempts, startup costs, risks, and lack of guarantees. In spite of these barriers, mergers are a viable alternative to selling to a hospital.

Mergers too often fail because they are approached the wrong way. Hiring a lawyer is the first thing most groups do when they decide to explore a merger. Lawyers don't "explore," they document.

The first step in merging with like-minded groups is exactly that—find like-minded groups. Single-specialty mergers are easier because physicians in the same specialty likely face the same challenges in their practices. For example, a couple of years ago I helped 30 pediatricians in eight groups explore a merger. It was fun to watch the camaraderie they established because they all faced the same problems unique to pediatrics.

Another thing I find in working with physicians on mergers is that their relationship with physicians in their specialty is often on a superficial professional level. Merging means going into business with one another, and the merger process is important because it allows physicians to get to know one another outside of a clinical setting.

One question that always comes up when creating a new group through merger is the question of size. How big should we be? How big do we need to be to impact payor contracting, add new services, or hire a professional manager?

The answer is: It depends. I have helped form several physician groups through mergers of more than 50 physicians. Some of those groups were extremely successful; others were only marginal successes because they failed to coalesce as a group and execute their business strategy.

The success of a merger is determined after the merger. It is driven by how well the new group executes its strategic plan. I have seen primary care groups as small as five affect payor rates and add profitable new services such as CT scanners to their offices. I have seen groups five times that size have little or no success with the same endeavors.

After you have identified like-minded colleagues to explore a merger, the next step is to find an experienced merger consultant. This is not as easy as it sounds. Every consultant and CPA firm working with physician practices will tell you they have experience in mergers. Take these claims with a grain of salt. Having once had one client who merged with another practice doesn't qualify as real experience in practice mergers.

Ask for references of groups of similar size and take the time to talk to the physicians about their merger experience. An experienced merger consultant will be glad to provide you with a list of questions and discussion points.

Successful mergers have a good foundation. Your merger consultant should take you through discussions of your purpose, vision, motivations, and fears. The consultant should complete a detailed financial assessment of each practice. You should also expect to spend a lot of time talking (without lawyers) about how you want to govern yourselves and manage your business.

Financial projections should be prepared combining all of the practices into one entity and overlaying changes that will be made as a result of the merger.

Avoid merger consultants who tout economies of scale as one of the big benefits of a merger. This, more than anything, shows a lack of experience. In most mergers, costs go up, at least initially and often permanently. This is because typically you are hiring a higher level of management and creating the management infrastructure necessary to manage a larger organization. Staffing cuts and other cost-cutting measures often do not materialize.

I have been involved in dozens of mergers involving hundreds of practices, and I have rarely seen overhead go down. Yet in spite of this increased overhead, I have seen revenue and physician incomes go up, often substantially, in a vast majority of mergers.

If overhead is projected to go down, make sure you have specifics. Which offices will be closed, which staff (by name) will be cut, and what other specific costs will be eliminated? It is easy to talk about cutting overhead in generalities, but it becomes much more difficult when you are forced to examine it at a detail level.

One area where practices can gain some economies in a merger is in the area of capital purchases. A good example is in IT. Major economies can be gained in sharing the cost of practice management, billing, and EHR systems.

Another example is in shared ancillary service development such as the CT services mentioned earlier. The risk of buying a refurbished CT scanner for $100,000 may sound daunting to a solo or small group, but sharing the cost (and risk) among 10 physicians is much more palatable.

Once you have examined the finances, you should have a firm idea of the potential financial downside. The decision usually comes down to how confident you are that this downside can be made up with additional revenue.

You are ready to hire an experienced merger attorney once you can answer the following questions:

1. What are the purpose, vision, and mission of the group?
2. How will the group govern itself, make decisions, resolve conflicts, and manage day-to-day operations?
3. What is the projected overhead for the first year post-merger?
4. How will the group divide income, and what is the projected post-merger income for each physician in the group?
5. What are three or four specific things the group plans to do in the first 12 months to increase revenue and by how much?

An experienced merger attorney will guide you through translating all the decisions you have made into formal legal language.

While the legal documents are being drafted, your merger consultant will take you and your staff through the operational implementation of the merger. This involves working through the myriad detailed operational decisions that must be made prior to the merger effective date.

You should generally allow six months or so for this operational implementation process. The caveats mentioned in Chapter 9 apply—don't get caught up in an artificial timetable to "get the deal done." The list of issues can be broadly categorized as follows:

- Provider numbers and payor credentialing;
- Staff issues including employee benefits, personnel policies, etc.; and
- Accounting and finance.

While the task of merging can be overwhelming at times, it has many potential rewards: a practice with your chosen like-minded colleagues that allows you to retain you autonomy and operate in a business model you designed specifically to meet your needs.

CONSIDER AN ALTERNATIVE PRACTICE MODEL

Physicians who are skeptical of working for a hospital but unsure they can continue to face the difficult realities of the typical Medicare and commercial insurance-based private practice model may want to consider alternative practice models. Some of these models, such as concierge, retainer-based, and direct-pay practices, typically are suitable only for primary care physicians, but others may have some appeal to specialists as well. These models are increasingly emerging in many parts of the country.

The ACA, in some ways, hastened the development of these alternative practice models. The promise that healthcare reform would provide access to health insurance for an additional 25 million uninsured turned out to be (mostly) true. Unfortunately, for both providers and patients alike, the term "insurance" didn't turn out to be what many expected. A vast majority of this "new" health insurance coverage turned out to be high-deductible plans with correspondingly high co-insurance, providing insurance coverage for major health issues but often not a plan that actually pays for most routine care.

As discussed in Chapter 2, these high-deductible plans actually decreased cash flow in many cases, while adding billing complexity and making it more difficult to monitor and collect patient balances. For example, many of these new plans limited or even eliminated coverage for office visits subject to the simple copayment—a system most physician offices had become used to collecting and managing. Applying office visit charges to the patient's deductible leaves the physician's staff responsible not only for collecting 100% of the allowable charge directly from the patient, but also having to navigate and understand the literally dozens of varying plan terms and provisions.

In addition, in spite of promises "you can keep you doctor," commercial insurers were allowed to develop "narrow networks" of providers. Many of these networks offered such low rates of reimbursement that many physicians simply opted not to join. This system is driving both the patients and physicians to alternative models.

The affluent pre-Medicare-age baby boomer demographic is a prime target for these practices. For a typical monthly fee of $150 to $200, the patient gets same day or next day appointments that are much longer than the typical 15 minutes. They feel they have the attention of the physician who isn't rushing out to the next exam room. A typical concierge physician sees 8 to 10 patients per day and has a patient base of only about 600 patients compared to 2,500 to 3,000 in a typical primary care practice. The result is happier physicians and patients.

The math works too. A typical primary care physician in private practice collects about $500,000 per year before overhead. A typical concierge physician with 600 patients paying $2,000 per year would collect $1.2 million—more than double. Many concierge physicians are part of a concierge practice firm such as MDVIP, Paladina, Qliance, and MedLion. These firms can take as much as 33% of the revenue to provide administrative support, marketing, and other assistance in establishing and maintaining the concierge practice. That still leaves the physician with $800,000—a significant increase in revenue. In addition, it is likely that overhead will be reduced because much of the billing functions are reduced or eliminated as well.

These models not only allow the physician to spend more time with each patient and offer same- or next-day appointments, but the physician can get to know the patient and help with the patient's wellness too. While critics lament the likelihood that concierge practices will hasten the shortage of primary care physicians, what did they expect when the healthcare system is allowed to continually devalue primary care physicians?

The biggest risk in establishing a concierge practice is in attracting the 600+ patients who are willing to pay the $2,000 or so per year. Long-standing patients may feel abandoned and some backlash should be expected. Some transition of the care of long-standing patients may be necessary and the expertise of the above companies may be worth the cost to obtain their expertise in navigating these types of issues.

A careful assessment of the age and income demographics of the population in your service area and a sound marketing strategy are prerequisites to a successful concierge practice. There are also legal hurdles that need to be navigated in establishing concierge practices that can vary from state to state, so experienced legal counsel should be consulted before moving in this direction.

There are many additional alternative models that can be considered. For example, many commercial insurers are heavily promoting telemedicine, which can supplement income for a physician during down time or provide a flow of patients with minimal overhead. Specialists can consider an on-call practice, where they see consults or pre/post-operative patients in a primary care office and maintain no physical office of their own. Micro-practices in which physicians work out of one small room with little or no staff and physicians who work from a fully-equipped medical van and make house calls are some of the other alternative models we see in certain markets.

TAKEAWAY POINTS FOR CHAPTER 11

1. You may have endured a lengthy process and protracted negotiations and still have some nagging doubts. Review the reasons you originally decided to explore selling. Will the proposed deal likely solve these problems and meet your needs?
2. Make a list of your concerns with the proposed sale. Are the reasons quantitative or qualitative? Qualitative issues usually are much more important than quantitative ones when it comes to long-term satisfaction.
3. If the fit seems right but the hospital's offer simply isn't adequate, consider intermediate options. These include leasing your practice to the hospital, a PEM, or an MSO. Each of the options has pros and cons, but each lacks the same level of permanence of an outright sale, so one of these options may make it easier to test the waters.
4. An MSO can ease a majority of the day-to-day management burdens and afford you the opportunity to try out the hospital's ability to manage your practice without taking the full step of selling.
5. If you decide that remaining independent is the best course of action, you should have gained a good objective assessment of your practice by following the steps in Chapter 3.
6. You can continue down your current path or make some hard decisions. The biggest barrier to change is always the effort required to break habits and take risks.

7. If you decide to stay independent, you may need to incur debt to invest in your practice's growth. Consider engaging an outside consultant to work with your group to develop a comprehensive strategic plan, take the emotion out of these decisions, and keep you pointed in the right direction.

8. Consider merging with an existing larger group. Don't be scared off by past reputations or ancient history. Initiate discussions and go through the process—you might find a better fit.

9. When investigating a larger group, you are looking for group's physicians' incomes to be materially higher than yours because ultimately their incomes represent your potential income post-merger.

10. The biggest potential prize in joining a large group is often in the payor contracts. The success of the group's contracts should be evident by looking at the physicians' income levels.

11. Merging with like-minded colleagues is a viable alternative to selling to a hospital. While the task of merging can be overwhelming at times, it has many potential rewards: a practice with your chosen like-minded colleagues that allows you to retain your autonomy and operate in a business model you designed specifically to meet your needs.

12. Consider alternative practice models such a concierge, retainer-based, and direct-pay models in primary care and on-call practices for specialists. Micropractices, house call practices, and telemedicine are some of the other models that many physicians are exploring.

Checklist 1: Checklist for Taking Your Practice to the Next Level

Take the information and insight you've gained by going through the hospital sales process to chart a different course. Here are questions to help you get an overview of where you stand and where you may want to go:

1. What did you learn about your practice's finances (Chapter 3) that you can improve?

2. Why was your valuation (Chapter 5) less than you had expected ? What can you do to improve it?

3. What should be in your strategic plan to either make your practice a better candidate for sale in the future or make it thrive without the need to sell? Options could include the following actions:
    - Incurring debt to invest in ancillary services or technology;
    - Recruiting new physician associates or midlevel providers;

- Hiring a highly qualified (and highly paid) professional manager; and
- Becoming more creative and proactive about promoting your practice.

4. Consider whether your practice has stagnated for any of following reasons and make notes. What action would need to be taken to correct the problems?
   - Aging providers who get comfortable with below-average income levels;
   - An entrenched practice manager (sometimes a spouse) whose skills haven't evolved with the needs of the modern-day practice;
   - An unwillingness to invest in experienced management and billing personnel;
   - An aging patient base and/or deteriorating payor mix;
   - Fear of taking risks in practice expansion through additional physicians, mid-level providers, or ancillary services;
   - Bad experiences with former physician partners, associate physicians, or mid-level providers;
   - Lack of a business plan or strategy to address such things as service niches, ancillary services, mergers, and satellite offices;
   - Poor payor contract rates and lack of data, expertise, and willingness to negotiate better rates, coupled with an unwillingness to terminate marginal contracts;
   - Behavioral issues or personality clashes in a group practice with one or more physicians; and
   - A group practice compensation plan that does not properly incentivize behavior.

Checklist 2: Merge with an Existing Larger Group

1. You will be asked to provide financial data on your practice, and you should expect the group to provide the same data to you.
2. The larger group's income is the key component in deciding whether to join the group. Compare the physicians' incomes to yours and to the MGMA benchmarks you reviewed in Chapter 3. Their incomes represent your potential income post-merger.
3. Have your CPA or practice consultant review the financial information provided if it seems too overwhelming to do yourself. If physicians' incomes are higher, you want to understanding why:
   - Do they work more hours?
   - Do they see more patients?
   - Do they offer more ancillary services?
   - How does their overhead compare to yours in terms of dollars and percentage?
   - What will happen to your overhead when you join them?

- Will your costs actually go up because they have higher staff salaries and benefit costs?
- Will your office be consolidated into one of their locations?

4. Does the group have a streamlined valuation process to purchase your assets? Use your knowledge from the hospital as a reference point to determine the reasonableness of the offer.

5. What is the larger group's predefined merger model? Review the asset purchase agreement, employment agreement, and buy-sell (shareholders) agreement.

6. Physician groups generally do not have guaranteed salaries and incentive compensation or bonus plans, so review the compensation (or income distribution) plan. This can be complex, so the group should provide you with:
   - A pro forma financial projection of how your practice would fit into the group's existing compensation plan; and
   - A fairly accurate estimate of what your income would be post-merger.

7. Will you be an equal owner in the group? Some larger groups, especially those with significant earnings streams coming from ancillary services, may not be willing to offer a newly merged physician a full share of those ancillary profits initially. This may be reasonable, depending on your specialty and the types of ancillaries involved.

8. Look for a restrictive covenant. A physician group is not really a group without some glue holding the physicians together. If people can leave at any time whenever a decision doesn't go their way, the group isn't sustainable.

9. The buy-sell (or shareholders) agreement is an agreement among all of the partners and provides how physicians join (buy) and leave (sell) ownership in the practice. Generally the stock buyout will be a share of the value of the assets of the group. Be wary of buy-sell agreements that provide for excessive buyout payments, deferred compensation, and other provisions for payments to physicians no longer practicing.

10. The group probably will not be able to share specific information with you on its payor contracts before completion of the merger because doing so may constitute illegal price fixing. Ask questions about its contracting expertise and abilities. The success of the group's contracts should be evident by looking at the physicians' income levels.

11. Shy away from a group where everyone is not an equal shareholder with an equal vote in the affairs of the group. Group practices owned or controlled by

one physician or even a small group of "insider" physicians are generally not sustainable.

12. Also stay away from groups with physician incomes lower than yours.

13. Will you feel disenfranchised in larger groups because participation in governance is limited to board members? Or will you feel relief in not having to be involved in the day-to-day decision making? Is committee membership an option or an obligation?

Checklist 3: Merge with Like-Minded Colleagues

1. Hire a lawyer after you have explored options. Lawyers don't "explore," they document.

2. Find like-minded groups or physicians. Single-specialty mergers are easier because physicians in the same specialty likely face the same challenges in their practices.

3. Find an experienced merger consultant. Ask for references of groups of similar size, and take the time to talk to the physicians about their merger experience. An experienced merger consultant will be glad to provide you with a list of questions and discussion points.

4. With all parties, discuss your purpose, vision, motivations, and fears. Discuss how you want to govern yourselves and manage your business.

5. Each practice provides a detailed financial assessment. Financial projections should be prepared combining all of the practices into one entity and overlaying changes that will be made as a result of the merger.

6. Do not expect automatic "economies of scale." In most mergers, costs go up, at least initially and often permanently. You are typically hiring a higher level of management and creating the management infrastructure necessary to manage a larger organization.

7. If overhead is projected to go down, make sure you have specifics. Which offices will be closed, which staff (by name) will be cut, and what other specific costs will be eliminated? It is easy to talk about cutting overhead in generalities, but it becomes much more difficult when you are forced to examine it at a detail level.

8. One place to gain some economies in a merger is in the area of capital purchases, such as IT. Another possibility is in shared ancillary service development.

9. You are ready to hire an experienced merger attorney once you can answer the following questions:
   - What are the purpose, vision, and mission of the group?

- How will the group govern itself, make decisions, resolve conflicts, and manage day-to-day operations?
- What is the projected overhead for the first year post-merger?
- How will the group divide income, and what is the projected post-merger income for each physician in the group?
- What are three or four specific things the group plans to do in the first 12 months to increase revenue and by how much?

An experienced merger attorney will guide you through translating all the decisions you have made into formal legal language.

10. Operational implementation is the next step. This involves working through the myriad detailed operational decisions that have to be made before the merger effective date. You should generally allow six months or so for this operational implementation process with details such as the following:
    - Provider numbers and payor credentialing;
    - Staff issues including employee benefits, personnel policies, etc.; and
    - Accounting and finance.

Epilogue: Finding Your Home

The obituary of the private physician practice has been written many times. I remember pronouncements that "the era of private practice is dead" going back more than 20 years. Physicians are trained to be independent thinkers and to function with a high degree of autonomy, and that may be why private practice has endured so long.

While the hospitals' success in this wave of employment has not been determined, warning signs of failure are appearing. I used to think success would be driven by the hospitals' willingness and ability to transcend typical hospital-centric thinking (and politics) and try new models and approaches. Large organizations turn slowly, and sometimes change never comes. It isn't looking as promising as it did even a few years ago, and I see the same mistakes being made.

I wonder about the financial sustainability of many of the hospital-employed physician networks already in place. Hospitals continue to consolidate, but bigger isn't always better and healthcare is still local. Will the "new money" arrive in time and in sufficient levels to sustain them? Are hospitals really the best partners to be at the forefront of integrated networks in the first place? Are they really the right organizational structure?

The cultural divide between younger and older physicians has been widening for many years, and this will continue to make it extremely challenging for physicians in private practice to recruit and sustain their business models as baby boomer physicians retire. I do not think private practice is dead, but I think it needs to evolve.

Some physicians are disillusioned with private practice and reconciled to making the best deal they can with the hospital. Others are disillusioned with hospital employment and are terminating their employment and reestablishing private practices. Yet many successful private physician groups continue to thrive in both single and multispecialty models.

These physician practices can and will continue to survive over the coming years without being part of an integrated system. There will be many opportunities and options for them to participate in the new payment models as independent practices or they will create their own. Many ACOs that are being created by large medical groups and even hospital systems will find success. Patient-centered medical home participation is often facilitated by commercial payors, and that may be an option too. New models will emerge.

If you are skeptical about selling, move with caution. You may face huge challenges if you sell and it doesn't work out. Reestablishing a private practice is difficult and risky. Unless your retirement is imminent, selling your practice at this stage in the cycle should be pursued only by carefully considering a possible exit strategy if needed.

Review the options in Chapter 11,because it explores some of the non-hospital options such as mergers and joining a larger group that are often overlooked as options.

www.ingramcontent.com/pod-product-compliance
Lightning Source LLC
Chambersburg PA
CBHW081539220326

41598CB00036B/6491